E. Marguerite Lindley

Health in the home;

A practical work on the promotion and preservation of health, with illustrated prescriptions of Swedish gymnastic exercise for home and club practice

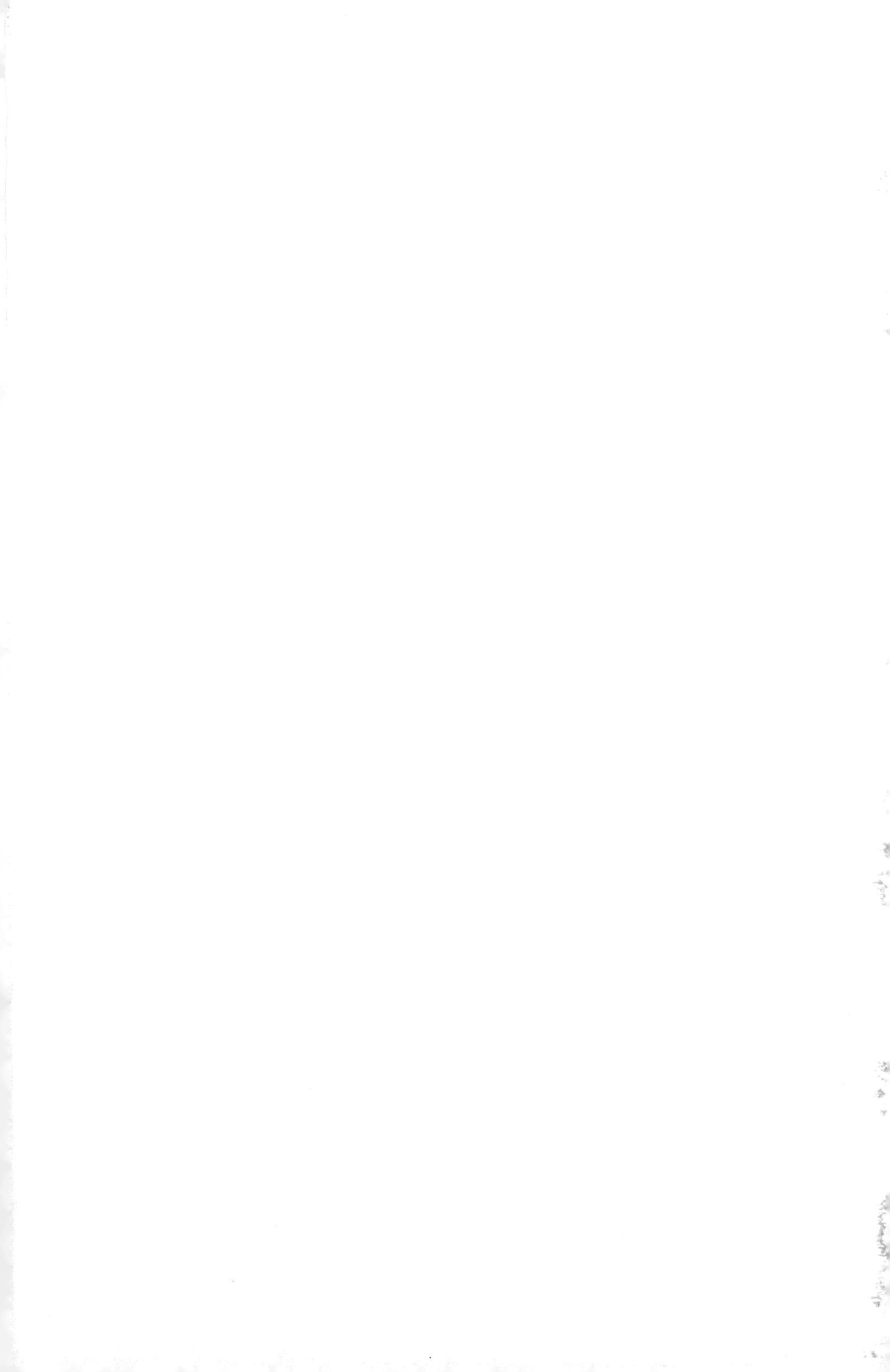

E. Marguerite Lindley

Health in the home;
A practical work on the promotion and preservation of health, with illustrated prescriptions of Swedish gymnastic exercise for home and club practice

ISBN/EAN: 9783337724061

Printed in Europe, USA, Canada, Australia, Japan

Cover: Foto ©ninafisch / pixelio.de

More available books at **www.hansebooks.com**

HEALTH IN THE HOME

A PRACTICAL WORK ON THE

PROMOTION AND PRESERVATION OF HEALTH

WITH ILLUSTRATED PRESCRIPTIONS OF

SWEDISH GYMNASTIC EXERCISE FOR HOME AND CLUB PRACTICE

BY

E. MARGUERITE LINDLEY

LECTURER ON HEALTH-CULTURE

NEW YORK
PUBLISHED BY THE AUTHOR
MURRAY HILL HOTEL
1896

Press of J. J. Little & Co.
Astor Place, New York

TO MY SISTER

WHO HAS PROVED THE VALUE OF THESE THEORIES ON PRACTICAL HYGIENE, SWEDISH MOVEMENTS AND MASSAGE, BY DAILY PRACTICE WITH HER CHILDREN DURING THE TWELVE YEARS OF HER MOTHERHOOD

I DEDICATE THIS BOOK

CONTENTS

CHAPTER XVII

CHAPTER XVIII

CHAPTER XIX

CHAPTER XX

CHAPTER XXI

CHAPTER XXII

CHAPTER XXIII

CHAPTER XXIV

CHAPTER XXV

PREFACE

"Our lives are albums written through
With good or ill, with false or true;
And as the blessed angels turn
The pages of our years,
God grant they read the good with smiles
And blot the ill with tears."

—WHITTIER.

THIS work is written at the request of many earnest women who realize the great need among our people of a better knowledge of the body and of the natural laws that govern it, and who realize that such knowledge can come only through physical education in the home. Most of the ills that afflict the human body are the outgrowth of insufficient knowledge of one's self; and, in this my first volume, I shall lay a foundation of such knowledge as will go far toward teaching self-preservation, the prevention of invalidism, both physical and mental, and the restoration to our people of their birthright of health.

No one chapter is independent of the others. They form together a system of primary instruction intended as a base for broader reading and study. I have avoided technicalities. This book is not intended as a text-book on anatomy, physiology, and hygiene. It is one of rational suggestions for health culture in the home and the school. We have able writers on the science of health, but not one on practical self-preservation, which is my aim in this volume.

No effort has been spared to make the work accurate, and I have inclined toward the safe side in advice where there could be the slightest doubt of accuracy. I submit the book with no misgivings as to its absolute safety and practical utility. If it leads any one to more extensive self-study, or to follow out the instructions contained in its pages, its mission will be complete.

In sending this volume upon its mission of life, I desire to gratefully acknowledge my obligations to the different writers whose ideas I have endeavored to follow. The book is based largely upon the writings of Claës J. Enebuske, Baron Nils Posse, Hartvig Nissen, and Dr. Edward Mussey Hartwell, in their works on physical education and Swedish gymnastic exercise; Gray's "Anatomy," and Potter's "Quiz on Anatomy;" and Dr. Yeo, Landois and Stirling, and Michael Foster on physiology. Hare's "System of Practical Therapeutics" contains contributions of great value, by Dr. I. Burney Yeo, on "Nutrition and Foods;" Dr. Simon Baruch, on "Hydro-therapy;" and Dr. Benjamin Lee, on "Massage."

Most of the chapters have been submitted to the able criticism of Dr. Yeatman Wardlow of New York, whose aid has been invaluable, through his large and successful experience in diseases peculiar to women.

The children who have posed for the pictures have never had access to the gymnasium, and not even the advantage of school gymnastics, but have followed prescription exercises, under their mother's supervision, as bed-time practice. Although of delicate tendencies, their development of health and figure are faultless, except in the case of the child whose spine shows curvature. This curvature was the result of a fracture of the arm, and has already almost disappeared under careful massage and exercise. It was purposely exaggerated somewhat for the picture, and there will soon be no trace of it left. This should be an encouragement to children, and should stimulate mothers to follow out similar home practice exercises with their own children.

E. MARGUERITE LINDLEY.

NEW YORK, *Jan.* 28, 1896.

HEALTH IN THE HOME

CHAPTER I

THE BODY A MACHINE

"The proper study of mankind is man."—POPE.

DESCARTES says: "If it be possible to perfect the human race, it is in medicine we must seek the means;" and explains that the term *medicine* is used in its broadest sense, as a science devoted to care of the body.

The body as a machine is less understood by the mysterious being styled the individual than is any other feature of evolution or creation that has yet come into our possession. Except in rare cases, it has been so mysterious a presence that no one but medical authorities have been allowed to fathom it. Indelicacy has been the apology for rearing past generations in dark ignorance of themselves; and, even now that the dawn of intelligence seems near, it is still considered necessary by many parents and teachers that an impenetrable wall of propriety, adjusted, in ages past, through mistaken ideas of civilization, admitting no daylight beyond respiratory, circulatory, and digestive organs, shall stili remain, and that the youth of both sexes must seek other instructors for a complete knowledge of their bodies, which it is their right to possess. We must now demand for the health of our rising generation a true knowledge of the body and mind, and of the laws that govern them, to supplant the wrong ideas that have grown out of the imperfect education formerly given, and consequent stolen information many have obtained from wrong sources.

The body was favorably introduced to the world a few years since by a sensible writer's calling it "the house we live in." That appellation seemed to break the ice. The remark found favor with thousands who had wondered what there was so mysterious about the body that it had been locked up from average ken all these generations, and they began to explore its hidden recesses.

It is certainly the dwelling place and vehicle of ego. It consists of a framework perfectly joined, covered with other building material, and spaced off into cavities; each cavity is furnished with a system of organs for use of the individual, whose throne is the brain. But the body is more than a house or a vehicle; it is a machine. According to the dictionary meaning of the term, we may understand the word machine as "a body used to transmit and modify force and motion; especially a construction consisting of a combination of moving parts, with their supports and connecting framework, by which power is applied or made effective, or a desired effect produced." This covers all the possibilities of the body, except the element life, and the definition of this word is yet beyond all human power.

The body is divided into four cavities—cranial, chest, abdominal, and pelvic. Each contains an individual system of organs that is of itself independent, working its purposes for the individual, yet entirely dependent on other systems of organs, and having no functional power if isolated from the others. The body itself expresses the functional unit made up of the many systems.

The body is often called "the human engine," and as such we had best consider it, except that it is possessed of organism and needs rest; while cleanliness, fuel, and water cover the requirements of the inorganic engine. An engine seems almost to possess intelligence. It eats and drinks, and converts the resources thus gathered into force, which is generated by combustion and supported by oxygen. The human engine is still more wonderful. Organs more intricate than those of the internal structure of the steam engine work ceaselessly night and day, through sickness and health, converting food and drink into force, which is generated by combustion and dependent upon oxygen.

The human engine is composed of a framework of bones, fastened at movable points by sinews, ligaments, and muscles which are controlled by the individual. We speak of such as voluntary muscles. The internal organs are controlled by involuntary muscles; but, like the voluntary, they are of and for the individual. Nerves are the mediums between mind and matter.

The nervous system consists of brain, spinal cord, and nerves. The brain consists of gray matter and white matter. The gray matter is the seat of manufacture of nerve power; the white matter is continuous with the nerves, which are the messengers through which sensation is made thought, and thought is made action.

The brain is divided into the cerebrum, the seat of intellect—or perhaps we had best say the individual—and the cerebellum, the seat of finer coördination.

Ganglia are supply stations of gray nerve matter, located at convenient intervals, so that the nerves may gain force other than from the brain direct. Important among them are the chains situated on each side of the spine, extending its entire length, and known as the sympathetic nerve system. It controls involuntary muscles and internal organs.

Without nerve force we are devoid of all power, and nerve force is entirely dependent on power obtained from the functions of the organs controlled by the nerves. This emphasizes the remark that the body is the functional unit. We speak of paralysis when nerve action is in some way or to some extent impaired. It is not a condition of weak muscle tissue, but lack of power in the nerve centres that control the affected muscles, or some lesion in the course of the nerves themselves. We improve the conditions by stimulating the circulation, either by means of passive exercise (as massage) or electricity, and by this means the nerve centres will gain strength, providing complications are not serious, and influences of an unfavorable nature do not overrule the good results of the treatment.

CHAPTER II

ON PHYSICAL TRAINING

"My people are destroyed for lack of knowledge."—HOSEA.

PHYSICAL training is a subject which has been forcing itself more and more upon the attention of American people for many years, not only because of the increasing popularity of athletic sports, to which it necessarily appertains, but also because a conviction has grown up in thoughtful minds that it is an essential to correct living.

The object of physical training is twofold—health of mind and of body—and the last must be first. Now, as in the old days of Greek glory, the development of the perfect physical type should be considered more important than mental training, since mental vigor is based wholly upon physical resources. But we will consider both as well-fitting halves of a balanced whole, and refer to the body as a unit consisting of these two parts.

Health is dependent upon laws which govern

the body; and the physical condition of the individual depends largely upon his knowledge and observance of these laws.

It is therefore most important that he should know himself; that he learn the anatomy and chemistry of his own body—the curious and wonderful structure as a whole, and the various organs, tissues, and component parts severally, in their individual use, and in their relation to each other, and to the entire mechanism of the human form.

One having this knowledge of the structure and use of the body will realize the necessity for harmony of strength, and will strive to develop and conserve, not dissipate, his forces.

Having established health, he is then equipped and fortified for longevity in its completest sense, and for a useful and noble career.

The body is trained by exercise of the voluntary muscles in obedience to the will, and such exercise must be regulated by a thorough knowledge of the influence they are likely to exert, not only upon the muscles, but upon the internal organs and the nervous system.

Bodily development, good posture, and flexibility of muscle are all essentials of ideal health;

but muscular power is by no means of paramount importance, as the athlete might insist.

To be sure, practice of certain movements recommended in this book is calculated to increase strength of muscle, but that is only a secondary consideration; the chief aim is to promote health of the internal organs and flexibility of muscle.

Enebuske, an eminent Swedish authority on movements, says: " Those who labor to enrich the muscles only, often make piteous beggars of the heart and lungs. Theory and experience show that a system of training may be followed which, while it develops muscular strength to a considerable degree, at the same time causes dilatation of the heart and lung cells, consequently making their walls thinner and weaker. Upon such training common sense stamps the seal of disapproval."

It is unnecessary for a man to be able to support a piano on his chest to demonstrate good lung power. Such phenomenal strength is rarely possible, and never necessary in physical training. Neither do horseback riding and the more vigorous work of rowing, bicycling, etc., or one-side games, as tennis and croquet, take the place of any systematic physical training; and in many instances these are not even desirable recreations for women and girls. In any case they should only be indulged in with moderation, as hygienic diversions, by those of good pelvic health. Women and girls need rational physical exercises, arranged to meet their individual conditions and requirements, for the development of unused muscles, and for strengthening their internal organs.

Too much stress cannot be laid upon the vital importance of having such a course of exercises intelligently prescribed. There was a time when all miscellaneous motions possible to the human being were accepted as physical culture. The teacher of such "exercises" held her own through the dark days of fads, by posing gracefully, and showing movements, unexplained, which her pupils imitated without understanding, and which were a caricature of the noblest of arts—body building. To meet the present demand for skilled labor, whether of the hand or brain, the director of physical culture must now be prepared by a course of study not inferior to that required for a medical *diplôme*. The knowledge of anatomy, physiology, psychology, therapeutics, dietary, practical hygiene, and emergency work is as indispensable to a proper application of the means of physical culture in relation to the vital and other internal organs, to defective organs, and to complications of defects, as it is to the physician in his study of the relation of drugs to health and disease.

One needs as thorough an equipment for the responsible task of developing and preserving the health as does the doctor for his mission of healing the sick.

Self-knowledge should begin for the little child in the kindergarten. When he is taught about the spine of a leaf, let him at the same time learn of his own spine, and, similarly, of his organs and their functions, which correspond to the organisms of plants and flowers.

In this way comes a reverent comprehension of what life means; and the body is not a mysterious belonging, to be abused in ignorance and degraded by disease, but a beautiful part of the great, wonderful harmony of creation, which must sound no false note, create no discord. The little child has begun to respect himself.

Let a good foundation of organic health and muscular control be established by careful progressive training, and then gymnastical athleticism need not be the calamity which it often proves to our too-rapidly trained girls and men. This requires fuller explanation—such exercise should be reached by years of preliminary training. Instead, many enter the gymnasium for their first lesson, and seek to accomplish, at once, results which tax them too severely, thereby exhausting their powers to an extent which handicaps them for the rest of their lives, if it does not make them downright invalids.

It is the same sort of overstrain which, in our restless business and social life, is filling our homes and hospitals with invalids, and our institutions with insane and feeble-minded.

From the cradle to the grave proper care of the body should be the first consideration, and all other things desirable will then be added.

Fresh air, correct diet, systematic exercise, hygienic bathing and dressing, and a sufficient amount of rest are the basis; these, if instilled from infancy, may become second nature.

That our ancestors seemed to do quite well without paying any special heed to such matters, can be no argument for us in this age of rapid, exhaustive living; yet it is not doubted that if they had lived more rationally, the present generation would be much better off. Had they cared wisely for bodily health and development, their descendants would not so easily succumb to the influence of colds, fatigue, contagion, and the encroachments of disease as they now do, and they would have more resistive power, greater staying power, and an all-round better physical heritage.

Heredity and environment are strong names to conjure with; but it is wonderful how far they may be controlled, and their influence obviated, through a rational comprehension of them, and by means of applied physical training.

Heredity is more strongly traced in mental than in physical characteristics. Fortunately, physical defects are transmitted as tendencies only, and inheritance of disease is rarely possible. From successive generations of unhygienic living, tendencies to certain diseases have been handed down, and they in turn have developed into actual disease, for want of a strict observance of the laws of health on the part of the descendants. This has been long looked upon by the hopeless victims as an inevitable law of heredity, which has been fulfilled by a dispensation of Providence, either in grudge or punishment for some sin of our ancestors—as if Providence ever generated an individual merely to consign him to a useless career, or an early and painful death!

Weak conditions of body or of mind are visited upon successive generations not as a punishment, but as the consequence of abuse of nature's laws; and these consequences may be to a great degree mitigated, and occasionally averted, if the operation of physical laws and of environment be made as careful a study as are the various mental sciences.

Again let me urge, know thyself. Study from the best accepted authorities the structure of the human body, the use of its many organs, their relation to one another, the harmony of their functions. Learn how to use, and, what is of equal importance, how to rest the body; how to feed, clothe, and bathe it. Ascertain the amount of its reserve force, and then keep a nicely adjusted bank account of resources and expenditures, and you will find it possible to balance the disadvantages of unfavorable heredity, and to adjust your environment to the end of health, longevity, and happiness, exceeding, no doubt, that of the individual who boasts more favorable heredity.

We crave length of days only when our powers are well preserved; when the body is exhausted, and we are doomed to drag out existence, a slave to infirmity and disease, living becomes labor and sorrow, and it is a release to pass away.

The physical ailments most common among American people are consumption, catarrh, rheumatism, scrofula in its various forms, neuralgia and other nerve diseases, and indigestion—the root of most of our bodily ills. It would be wiser to aim for the prevention of these maladies than to wait until they are present, and then seek their cure. If taken in their incipiency, their cause ascertained, and their conditions subjected to as skilful and faithful treatment as is acute suffering, in the majority of instances the enemy might, even if not wholly routed, be at least kept at bay for many happy, useful years of the victim's lifetime.

It is too common a practice to disregard the signs of approaching disease until its development is too far advanced to be controlled, and then to bemoan "the hand of Providence," which has laid the sufferer low. It is not Providence; it is ignorance and neglect and custom. They, especially custom, which underlies the whole fabric of our physical, social, and, alas, also our spiritual lives, are responsible. Custom has for a long time overlooked the necessity for education of the body, and, therefore, except in rare cases, experience and observation have had no chance to argue. A woman beholding frail health resulting from imprudence in others, will still persist in her own similarly imprudent ways, not reasoning that she must surely be called to account for these wrongs done the flesh—wrongs that may not revert to her personally, but cannot fail to be visited upon her children. This is not her fault, it is merely her misfortune in having followed customs that are unhygienically adjusted.

Parents continually do their children the great wrong of mistaking the true aim in their education—physical perfectness. They do not realize that a child is only fortified for intellectual adult life when health is so thoroughly established that no concessions need be granted to ills or ailments. Instead, they struggle to equip their offspring with overcrowded brains, toppling above weak, poorly developed bodies, and education is for them a sort of incubating process.

The strength of every nation depends upon its women, and this strength emanates from the home. How, then, can men live and thrive when the women that make those homes are semi-invalids? What can be expected for the future when we see only frail, emotional girls being reared to fill the places of the present generation of delicate women? For men not properly reared are a discredit, a dishonor, to the women whose influence shaped their lives. "The woman's cause is man's. They rise or fall, dwarfed or god-like, bond or free. If she be ill-shaped, how can men thrive?"

CHAPTER III

EARLY LIFE AND TRAINING OF CHILDREN

"The child is father of the man."—WORDSWORTH.

THIS chapter would probably better claim attention of the progressive woman were it headed "Heredity and Environment;" but for the practical, every-day suggestions it contains, this simpler title seems preferable. Heredity is too broad a subject to find foothold in any introductory volume on health preservation, and in this it will be mentioned only as a guide-post to posterity. We will consider environment as an influence possible of adjustment for weal or for woe, and, confining the argument within these limits, allow the "sins of the ancestors" to rest with their bones.

The environment of the child should be a leading study with women. The child of to-day is the man or woman of the future, the law-maker and law-breaker of our country, and the responsibilities incumbent upon the rearing of that individual are enormous.

Holmes says: "The physical training of a child should begin two hundred years before it is born." While the truth of this is strikingly apparent on every hand, in the spectacle of undesirable citizens one meets every day, we will render the argument more practical and possible and near, by saying its training should begin two years before it is born. For the sake of propagating the highest types of our race, physically, mentally, morally, the parents themselves should be in the highest possible condition and possession of these. We have but to look into the history of crime, poverty, and imbecility to find this truth strongly emphasized.

In the present struggle for the advancement of women, let us not forget that woman's sphere is in the home, and that motherhood is her privilege, not her curse. Her life is not necessarily narrowed by a realization of these facts, however. She must broaden, not ignore, her sphere.

The mother's first duty is self-preservation, else she is but a poor altruist. In the execution of mistaken ideas of duty, her stamina is too often reduced to a pitiable stage. She should study to spare herself frivolous care.

What matter if Mrs. Grundy's house possesses a few more tinselled draperies, and the table is furnished with more bits of useless china than hers? She should possess the true moral independence which is conceded to American women, and live within her own conscience, if not always within her own desires. A plain house, a plain table, and plain clothing, if such are in accord with her resources of health, she would best accept, and not fritter away her vitality with care of frivolous belongings, such as her neighbor may be better able physically to superintend. Bodily health, freedom from excessive emotionalism, and a clear conception of real from mistaken duty, will preserve every mother from continued fatigue, except in emergency or misfortune. Some emotional women seem to consider it their fate to look tired, unmindful of their privilege and duty to keep as rested, fresh, and cheerful as possible. Let such women look into other homes, and observe the misery which results from invalidism of the mother, and they will be glad to strive to prevent it in their own case.

Specific physical training for the baby should begin from the first moments of his life, in the rational care given his little body. Dress, food, baths, and proper handling constitute the main features of this care.

Dress should be of light weight and of few pieces, so that baby is not disturbed to any extent by the process of dressing and undressing. His clothing should be of soft wool fabrics. These are seamless, porous, and elastic; sympathetic to the skin, neither overheating nor chilling it. Air should always be permitted to reach the child's skin and give its aid in promoting vigorous growth. Four Jersey wool garments constitute the baby's hygienic dress; viz., the knit abdominal band (this should be worn during at least the first ten years of the child's life, to prevent intestinal disturbances from cold), high-neck and long-sleeve shirt, sleeveless skirt made in one piece, and dress. The skirt may be placed inside the dress so that the two may be adjusted at one and the same time, or the shirt, skirt, and dress be arranged together for but one adjustment. Neither skirt nor dress should exceed three-quarters of a yard in length. Dainty mull gowns may be used outside these, to please the artistic eye, if desirable, but volume should be avoided. Baby, like any other little animal, is happiest and healthiest when his limbs are free. Stockings, not kick-off-able socks, constitute the leg and foot gear. What is known as the "Dorothy System" will be found very helpful to young mothers. The napkin should also be of soft Jersey wool, and should be gored and fitted to the shape of the hips and lower back. Too much bulk should not be allowed in this garment. Good authorities affirm that many cases of curvature, bow legs, ungainly posture, knock knees, pigeon toes, and awkward gait have their origin in its incorrect use.

The baby's diet is apt to be an experimental affair, and the conditions of mother and child are so necessarily varied that little can be said on general principles regarding it. Artificially fed children are more liable to disease than those nourished naturally by a healthy mother. Still, artificial feeding can be safely managed if proper care is observed.

Mothers often ask me regarding the different food preparations for infants. It is the physician's province, rather than mine, to recommend these, as he would decide from baby's conditions and tendencies what would be most nourishing and permanently beneficial. The decision is usually in favor of Lactated Food, or Mellin's Food, as a staple. The latter has been the longer on the market, but the former is quite on a par in general approbation. In many instances no other food is given during the first two years. Such food should always be at hand, to serve for adult as well as child, when the appetite refuses heavier nourishment. When dentition begins, hard breads of gluten, not graham flour, should be given the child. This is not entirely for nutrition, but to strengthen the organs of mastication as well. It should appeal to thinking mothers as a preventive of early loss of deciduous teeth, which we frequently find the case with children who are fed entirely on liquids and cereals.

The quantities of food allowed in any case should be moderate, and at intervals corresponding to the age and condition of the child. An able English writer says: "During the first month of a child's life there should be no fixed time for giving nourishment. In one of slow digestion the intervals should be longer than in one of more rapid digestion. The cry of hunger should be met with a moderate amount of food. Too large a quantity at any one time brings about malassimilation just as surely as deficiency of food does."

This fact should be impressed strongly on the mind of the indulgent mother. Her baby can be starved from overfeeding, by the digestive powers becoming overtaxed, and gastric juices wasted in consequent nausea. Give baby little sips of cold water sometimes when he clamors for what he doesn't really seem to need, and it will calm his restlessness quite as effectually as food will, and without harm.

Sir James Clark points out forcibly how imperfect nutrition from mismanagement of diet in the early days of life lies at the root, or very near the root, of the development of scrofula, consumption, and other diseases which appear in later years. Other authorities locate the germs of intemperance in the nursery, from overindulgence in eating, and consequent lack of self-control throughout the growing period and in adult life.

Bath habits should be adjusted from a rational comprehension of the use and abuse of bathing. (See chapter on Baths.) It is a great error to bathe the baby immediately after feeding. At least an hour should elapse before the bath. Baths should be given early in the day, before the first feeding, if possible. The little body is prepared for good results from its food, by having its circulation stimulated in this way.

Baby should never be allowed to grow chilled by his bath; have the room at suitable temperature; seventy-five degrees is a fair average for the healthy child. In cases of nervous or delicate children, bathe the body in sections, keeping all other parts covered, and covering what has been bathed before exposing more surface to the air. Or, bathe under a blanket, if necessary. The temperature of the bath should be gradually lowered from warm to tepid, as the age and condition of baby decide. Warm baths are not invigorating, and do not give firmness to tissues as tepid or cool baths do. If the warm bath is necessarily continued, follow it with massage (see chapter on Massage; also, Passive Work for Infants); this aids greatly in improving conditions of circulation, and had best always follow the bath until vigorous growth is established. The bath hour is a favorable one for moulding irregular features and for giving massage treatment for poorly developed muscles. (See chapter on Massage.)

While dressing, bathing, and holding baby generally, place his head towards the strong light, so that the rays do not strike his eyes. Observe this rule also in regard to sleeping. The bed should be a firm hair mattress. Occasionally alternate the infant's position from one side to the other during sleep. The right is the more favorable soon after a meal, as the stomach walls are less taxed in their efforts to digest the food from that posture than from the left side. It can be easily seen that the stomach is emptied from this position with less effort on the part of nature.

Rough, careless handling of a young baby often causes rupture or spinal defects, which may not give evidence of grave conditions until years afterwards. The baby should be handled as little as possible. He should be permitted to lie on his back and kick out his own preferred exercises. Trotting, joggling, and rocking must never be allowed. The perambulator is a valuable accessory to the nursery, but its limitations must be established. I will give a few suggestions. The baby's back should have a firm, straight support, and not be allowed to round out, as is usually the case when soft pillows are placed as props. The tissues easily shape themselves well or ill in these early months, and the physical environment of babyhood often decides the health of the adult. Baby must not be allowed to fall asleep in a sitting posture, and to be joggled from that drooping position, lest the spine suffer. Neither should he be placed on his back in the open air, with the glare of strong light falling upon his upturned face. Place him on his side, or else make sure that the canopy is well darkened with green. The mother should never trust him far or long beyond easy reach. Even the trustiest nurse sometimes forgets these important points, and harm may be done to eyes and spine which in after years will prove a barrier to success in the careers of valuable citizens. At best, too few of these little human machines stand the vital test called living, and the mother must watch well the influences brought to bear upon her little one, in order to prevent disaster from reaching him. Her reward is ample for the few years' sacrifice of other interests which this vigilance demands.

Shocks from fright must be spared the little ones, and clamor and confusion are injurious to their nerves.

Kissing the baby should not be allowed. The impure breath of adults may breed riot in his delicate organism, and disease germs are easily thus conveyed. The custom also causes nervousness. It would be objectionable to a healthy twelve-year-old boy, and should not be thrust upon the helpless baby. Such emotional ceremonies must be forbidden by intelligent mothers. These usages are certainly declining in popularity, which is fortunate for the babies. Train the child to allow visitors to kiss his hand.

Walking and sitting up should rarely be forced, should seldom need be encouraged, and should never be long continued. Massage and kicking are the best exercises for developing baby's strength.

The trials of dentition and actual illness should at once receive medical attention.

From the nursery to the school is a critical change. Natural existence, we may say, now ends, and a new era opens. A mother cannot follow her child there; she must needs trust him to new and foreign influences. She is indeed fortunate if he begins school life in a good kindergarten, or at least in a school class of but few numbers, where his individuality may be studied and respected, and his bodily and moral health considered. A few minutes' conversation with one of a coarser mind will often arouse a curiosity regarding vulgar utterances that poisons for all its future years the child-mind. He must, in time, meet elbow to elbow the coarser element, but let us hope that this will not be until after he has been trained to understand and obey higher laws, and is the better able to resist the effect of low influences. The mother must ever keep her child's confidence. She should not evade his questions, nor give him half an answer. Such will not satisfy him for long, and once finding that he has been deceived by his mother, he will the next time seek advice from other sources, usually coarser ones, as they evade none of his inquiries. How much better that the child learn about the production of the hen's egg from his parents than from the cook or hostler. The hatching of a chicken from an egg is a marvellous phenomenon to a child. Some mothers aid the inquiring child's intelligence in this direction, yet close the doors to facts touching the similar process in mammalia, giving ridiculous accounts of the origin of kittens and babies.

I was once visiting at a country home where

household pets of every description were domiciled. After being called upon to admire some downy little chickens, a bright five-year-old boy next showed me his kittens, saying, "The mother cat laid them all hatched out." That boy is now twelve years old, and his mind is as clean and wholesome as it was in his babyhood. No morbid curiosity has ever degraded it. His mother has always given him truth in answer to his inquiries, and to her, rather than to the coachman or the cook, he has gone for enlightenment. God bless such mothers! They will never have occasion to sigh over the immorality of their boys; for immorality is the outgrowth of ignorance, and that ignorance, nine times out of ten, comes from the mother's mistaken idea of her duty in such respects. I hold mothers in contempt whose religion is chiefly emotional, and reaches not out to wholesome, practical instruction for the callow minds given them to rear in knowledge, as well as in the fear and love of God.

Instruction about the body should begin in the kindergarten, and extend through the school period. Teacher and mother are gravely responsible for the sin and invalidism which grow out of self-ignorance in children. They should be taught to dread disease, deformity, and insanity. Pride of health and figure should be daily topics.

In managing children be even in discipline, firm, but not severe; and modulate the voice from sharp or harsh intonations.

Be always consistent. Do not send the nurse-girl to "see what Harry is doing, and tell him to stop it," which illustrates some mothers' idea of discipline. "Because I tell you so," is another common and culpable answer to give a child when he asks the why and wherefore of an order. The child's rights demand rational explanation. His ideas are to his mind as correct as are the mother's to hers. Let her make clear the reason of her demands, and she then makes a convincing appeal to the child's sense of justice.

"Jack, did you do this?" "Yes," says Jack. "Then I will punish you." And the next time Jack says "No," and escapes punishment. "Mary, don't ever let me see you do this again;" and Mary never does—if she can help being found out. These irrational manifestations of "discipline" grate upon ear and sense daily. They should be regarded by mothers as grave errors in duty. "Train a child's will, not break it," says Tolstoï. A child's rights must be respected. Always give him a hearing, and reason him out of his errors. If he is left to chafe under what he considers injustice, he will in time become indifferent, callous, and morbid. The air has always rung with precepts concerning the duty of children to parents; but that law was written by a stern parent, who forgot he had ever been a child. Like any and every other law, it is reactionary, and duty of parents to children is equally as serious and obligatory.

A child's fussiness always has its origin in some physical disarrangement. It may be malnutrition, irregular habits, or but faults in dress, such as a trodden-over heel, or clothing which binds; or, perhaps, merely the erratic demands of an overindulged mind. If there is lack of physical comfort, remedy it, and the child's temper will, as a result, improve.

It is a bad practice to call attention to a child's faults; instead of this, try to change the influences that are favorable to such. Never, under any circumstances, discipline a child in the presence of others, whether guests or servants.

The prodigy is rarely appreciated outside the family circle. The fire that burns so brilliantly at first, often runs to ashes long before the world has seen the flash. The child of slow but healthy mental development will make the brighter man. It makes a child appear to disadvantage to hear attention called to his clever sayings. Generally speaking, a visitor's hearing is good, and the child's wit is appreciated without aid of its mother's emphasis. Better praise the child for his erect spine and high chest than for his wit. He will then develop into the more interesting man.

The overindulged child is also unfortunate. The mother is gravely neglectful of her duty in this case. Oftentimes she wrecks the child's digestion by permitting his overeating of sweets, as sugar on his cereal, etc. It is unnecessary to begin such a habit. The food is more palatable without than with it, if the taste is but thus cultivated. The mother should not make remarks in the child's presence regarding her dislike for any food he needs. Overeating is sometimes injudiciously encouraged until the child is like Johnnie with the batter-cakes, who "wished he hadn't some he'd already got."

Allowing a child to come direct from the cold outer air and overheat himself by the fire is not wise. Keep him occupied in a cool part of the room until his body is comfortable, and he will not then desire greater warmth.

Substitute cold water for ice-water as a beverage at all times of year, and he will thrive better, and escape many ills that are induced by chilling the stomach. Cold water is a safe drink, but had best be boiled and bottled, to insure its freedom from disease germs.

Never allow a child to spend the night with a playmate; and if a playmate spends the night with him, give the little guest an apartment separate from that of your own child. Confidences at such times are apt to be exchanged which may lead to dire habits in after life. I know every mother thinks her own child too pure-minded to contaminate another, but she must remember that the other child may not be equally pure-minded.

Before the cigarette-smoking age is reached, teach that it is sinful physiologically, not morally. Illustrate it by stewing a cigarette in a little water, and showing the child how quickly the juice will kill a fly or an ant. Teach him the absorption of the poison into his blood from smoking, and there will be no desire to smoke. Self-preservation is uppermost in a child's mind. He only needs instruction. It is said that cigarette smoking among the Indians is proving the greatest of all disasters to their health.

The nervous child should be restrained from violent, long-continued play. Leg-ache should be met with proper attention, not regarded as the penalty of a growing child. The healthy child has no leg-ache, even though his growth is more rapid than that of the delicate one. There are no "growing pains." If a child complains of pain, investigate at once the cause.

During the growing period, early bed-time should be the rule, and the little folks should, if possible, retire in a happy frame of mind.

If a child is subject to night terrors, be patient with him. Undue mental excitement may cause these alarms, such as stories of murders, burglars, or ghosts. Sometimes a physical disturbance is the cause, as indigestion, constipation, or worms, dentition, distention of bladder, or too violent frolicking just before bed-time. A child should sleep comfortably clothed, rather than warmly covered. Wool fabric is best for bed-clothing. Train the child to lie with arms out of bed. It is the best posture for chest muscles, and little hands so placed will not wander where they should not.

Regarding beds, study suggestions given for infants—a firm hair mattress, a small hair pillow, if any, the head of the bed towards the strong light, and the room continually ventilated.

Children should not be taken into crowded places. Mothers had best not allow sight-seeing which involves this, until the little one's stature raises him above the stratum of foul air and the level of untidy clothing which is encountered in the average throng of miscellaneous humanity.

Fondling cats and dogs is also another unhygienic custom too often allowed children. The cat frequents localities where filth and disease germs lurk. These become imbedded in her fur, and then the child brings his little face close against kitty, to the serious detriment of health. Skin diseases are often conveyed in this way. The cat's breath is poisonous, and neither cats nor dogs can be relied on for selection of clean foods. This and the fact that the dumb brute's tongue is used in cleaning his body are, I trust, sufficiently convincing evidence that the mother should teach her child to allow no animal caresses on the face.

It is not wise to stand too heroically by the theories of our grandmothers in regard to the rearing of children. Their hearts were kind and their motives noble, but they had no scientific research upon which to found their theories, nor did they make the unfavorable results of their experiments a theoretic study for aid to others.

Had they systematized child-rearing to hygienic advantage, we of this generation would not be in the apologetic state of health we now are.

It is equally unwise to adopt the apparently successful experiments of others as infallible laws. Let such be merely suggestive of study, open to adaptation to the individual child. Remember there can be no universal laws for the rearing of children.

The first years of school life are most harmful to health. The regular habits already formed are apt to be disregarded. The morning bath is often neglected, and the morning and noon meals are taken too hurriedly. These two lapses alone produce physical discord, sooner or later. Better lose a half day of school than omit the morning bath. The physical health of the child is far more important than his mental progess, for that can be achieved later, while a ruined constitution is too often irretrievable.

Mother's clubs (or departments for this work in other clubs) should be established for the purpose of discussing and regulating school influences.

Bad posture threatens the little spine in early schooldays. Curbing the child's freedom in the matter of exercise, and keeping him in long-maintained sitting postures, are opposed to systematic development. Both at home and at school, chairs and desks are liable to be poorly adjusted to the conditions and needs of the young people. The girl suffers more than the boy from these inconveniences. Her spine is more flexible, and her body less bulky. She needs a lower chair and a higher desk than the boy does. (See chapter on Spine.)

These unfavorable influences should be met with good physical training, to encourage proportionate growth. Both gymnastic training and gymnastic games should form a leading feature of the school routine. The jerky work so disastrous to nerves, and the athletic tests so dangerous to heart action, as well as the meaningless posturing that is mere formulated motion set to music, for exhibitions, should never be tolerated. Let mothers see to it that so-called physical culture is not physical torture, and that the person directing it is well versed in the human machine and its requirements, and as thoroughly competent as is the mental educator to do her work.

Dr. Boulton, of England, fixes the average growth of children at from two to three inches per year, and says that a lesser growth than two inches, or more than three, should excite apprehension. Equally good authorities give a difference in individuals, however, as regards growth, due to conditions of nationality, climate, and environment of country or city living; but all agree that a falling below normal weight presages illness, and demands immediate attention.

We refer to such authorities as Drs. Enebuske and Hartwell of Boston, and Sargent of Cambridge, for data showing the working capacity and the resistance to fatigue of those trained in the gymnasium as contrasted with those receiving no such training, and for the height and weight of children as related to their age, and also to their power of resisting disease.

Too long continued concentration of mental forces upon any one subject is exhaustive rather than educative. The programme should be varied to avoid this, and in order to insure perfect mental digestion and assimilation.

Two or three hours of intellectual culture in the morning are too much for any delicate child, and as much as the robust child should be subjected to, up to the age of ten or twelve years. Let these few hours of mental application be followed by a rationally eaten meal, and then by an afternoon of wholesome outdoor life, and we shall not have the nervous, irritable children we now do. The average school-child eats his noon-day meal too rapidly, and hurries from it to play or study. Far better have no nourishment at that time other than a cup of broth, bovox, malted milk, or warm milk, if plenty of time for eating cannot be insisted upon.

The danger period is not past at sixteen; but, providing health of body and mind are well established, mental activity may then be forced, in proportion to physical resources, without much risk, but never should be strained beyond this point; good sleep and good digestion must on no account be impaired by mental effort.

The adolescent period is a most trying one. This extends, with boys, from the age of thirteen to twenty-four, and with girls from twelve to twenty-two approximately. The girl develops earlier than the boy, and her environment is less favorable than his, but her endurance is proportionately greater.

These facts should be taken into account when contrasting and carrying out their respective courses of study, for they afford a criterion of mental as well as physical training.

The boy suffers more than the girl from the mother's not explaining his physical development and consequent nervous conditions, and allaying the latter through hygienic measures and diversion. Discipline is not the remedy. Healthful surroundings for body and mind, self-reliance, self-control—these are the remedies.

On the other hand, the girl suffers more than the boy from her environment of dress and the oft-repeated admonition to be ladylike and not romp. She is in greater need than ever of fresh air and exercise, and is unable to understand, nor can her mother explain, why she is so suddenly denied the sports allowed her brother. She must not climb—her petticoats will show. She must not race nor jump about, because it is hoydenish. There is no way to meet this emergency but to dress the girl appropriately and let her romp and play. For underwear, she needs tights the color of her stockings; and skirts, if any are necessary, the color of her dress. Then running and climbing will bring no consciousness of hidden underwear revealed to the public. I repeat again, custom is the girl's worst enemy.

Emotional friendships, girl confidences, sensational literature, etc., are deadly enemies to the wholesome development of the intellect. Such must be anticipated and circumvented. Travel, botanizing, and other outdoor interests and occupations are helpful, though not all-sufficient; and a few minutes' return of unfavorable influence will ruin all beneficial conditions. Close, if possible, all avenues that admit such dangers.

During the early years of adolescence, and

possibly during the entire period, irregularities of nerve and physical health, weak eyes, troublesome ears and lungs, and morbidness of mind threaten. Meanwhile, habits of living should be carefully adjusted. Daily bathing, fresh air, wholesome food, comfortable clothing, plenty of sleep, systematized exercise, freedom from brain forcing—these are the considerations that must be observed in order to evolutionize the healthy, enduring individual.

Exercise, both systematized for uniformity of growth and generalized for diversion, should belong to school and college life. But neither one should ever, in the well-trained individual, be carried to excess. Bear in mind that exercise is of service in stimulating the circulation, and the circulation is the means employed for rebuilding and wearing off body-tissues, increasing respiratory power, augmenting activity of the skin, and thereby improving digestion, and regulating the kidneys and other functions of the body.

We are rearing our children to be the citizens of the times to come. They should be taught the Latin proverb, *Festina lente.*

CHAPTER IV

CIRCULATION

"I am fearfully and wonderfully made."

EVERY organized being is made up of what are technically known as tissues. Tissues are the different characteristic substances of the body, as, in the animal kingdom, bone, muscle, nerve, skin, walls of vessels, etc. They are composed of minute atoms which are continually undergoing a process of growth and destruction. This process of growth and destruction is effected, in the higher grades of animal life, through the blood, which carries the nutritive material of the food and the oxygen of the air to the different parts of the body, and also collects the effete or waste materials resulting from tissue change and combustion, and carries them back to the point of exit from the body.

The blood consists of a clear, pale fluid called plasma, which holds in suspension an enormous number of little orange-colored disks, about one three-thousandth of an inch in diameter, and a smaller number of larger colorless ones. These disks are called corpuscles. The orange-colored ones are called red corpuscles, as from the large quantities in which they are present in the blood they impart to it its red color. The colorless ones are called white corpuscles.

The corpuscles may be separated from the plasma by several methods at our command, which we have not space to describe here. If a drop of the plasma be placed upon the slide of the microscope, a curious change may be observed. Numerous delicate fibrillæ gradually interlace in a network somewhat resembling spider-web. These fibrillæ are called fibrin. The fluid remaining is called serum. This process is the cause of the phenomenon known as clotting, or coagulation. If blood is allowed to stand outside the body, this formation of fibrin soon results in transforming it into a semi-solid or jelly-like condition. The corpuscles then become entangled in the meshes of the fibrin, the serum oozes out, and the mass gradually solidifies.

This property of the blood is of the greatest consequence in stopping bleeding from injury, as the clot thus formed is nature's method of stopping a ruptured blood vessel. It will be further described in the chapter on Emergency Work.

The red blood corpuscles are greatly in excess of the white, a proportion in a healthy person of about three hundred to one. When the relative proportion of these is changed, the individual is not in condition of normal health. The red corpuscles contain the life-supporting and tissue-building elements. The color is from the element known as hæmoglobin, which is contained in the red corpuscles. The coloring element is of greatest importance in medico-legal work, and is a sure test of blood-stains, and, to a certain extent, also, of the age of the stains.

Illness, excessive fatigue, malnutrition, etc., exhaust the red blood corpuscles, and the white in turn are multiplied; hence the blood is, as we say, impoverished, and the individual is pale. Our first thought, then, is to build up the loss. This is best effected through rest, fresh air in abundance, and nourishing foods.

For the growth and repair of the body the blood absorbs elements from the foods we eat, and oxygen from the air we breathe, and distributes them throughout the body. It is wondrously interesting to know that each part selects its own building material from the blood, and that no part in the rationally fed and used system ever robs another part. The blood has another equally important use, that of removing waste matter—the refuse caused by activity of muscle, brain, etc.; or, as may be more clearly understood, by the destruction of tissues that accompanies body growth and repair. The refuse matter is known as carbonic acid gas, and is absorbed by the blood in place of oxygen, which is given off for tissue building. The color is changed from bright red to purple, and it is then designated as venous blood. Water is also added to the blood in the process. These undesirable elements are eliminated from the system through the functions of the lungs, kidneys, and skin.

The circulatory apparatus consists of heart, arteries, capillaries, and veins. The heart is a little muscular force-pump about the size of the fist, distinguished by the right and left sides, which, in the healthy person, are as two distinct organs, although working in unison. It is situated left of the centre of the chest, between the third and fifth ribs, inclined to the left, and backward, so that the right side is toward the front; but, on account of its unequal shape, the left ventricle is brought nearer

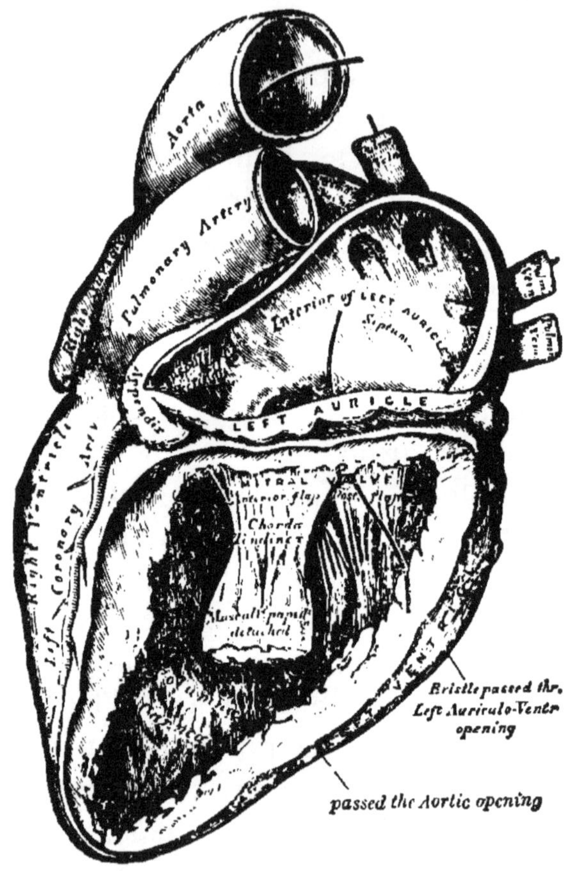

I.—SECTION OF LEFT SIDE OF HEART, SHOWING BLOOD-VESSELS THAT LEAD INTO AND OUT OF IT.

the chest walls. Each side is divided into two chambers, an auricle and a ventricle, which connect with each other by means of

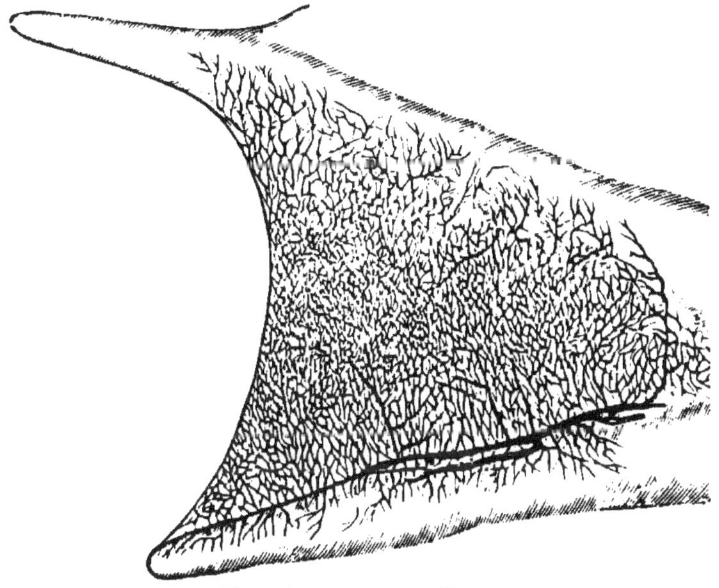

II.—Web-foot of a Frog.

For years the medical authorities knew of no blood-vessels other than arteries and veins, and were mystified as to what became of the blood between its leaving the terminal arteries and entering the corresponding veins, and what caused the change of color and quality. The existence of capillaries was finally discovered in the web-foot of a frog seen under the microscope.

an orifice, guarded by a tightly closing valve, opening into the ventricle from the auricle. The valves allow the blood to flow from the supply vessels into the auricles, from the auricles into the ventricles, and out of the ventricles, but not the reverse.

The arteries convey the blood sent outward from the heart to the tissues. Their walls are hard, and consist of three muscular coats. The middle one contains strata of "yellow elastic tissue," as it is called, which is a valuable agent in helping the heart in its work, by propelling the blood current in response to the heart-beat; this pulsation we detect in many localities, as at the wrist, and we speak of it as the pulse.

The capillaries are the connecting link between the last sub-division of the arteries and the smallest veins. They are exceedingly minute, about one three-thousandth of an inch in diameter, and through their walls the blood does its work. The tissues absorb nourishment and oxygen from the hæmoglobin of the blood, which enter into the growth and repair of the body, and the waste tissue is in turn absorbed by the blood, in form of carbonic acid gas, urea, and uric acid; the red color is thereby changed to purple, and the blood becomes venous. This is an important phase of the phenomenon we define as respiration, and completes the work of oxygenation by utilizing the oxygen obtained in the lungs.

The veins convey the return current of blood to the heart. They extend parallel with the arteries. Unlike the arteries, their walls are soft, and collapse on being emptied. The venous current is aided by muscular activity; the veins are also provided with valves which prevent the current from settling back in response to the laws of gravitation.

The rapidity of the blood current is of great interest. The complete circuit is made in from twenty to twenty-eight seconds; this velocity is much more marked in the arteries than in the capillaries.

Circulation is continuous; when there is cessation in any part we may look for disease. (See quotation from Dr. Lee, Chapter VIII., Swedish Exercises for the Home.)

Circulation comprises systemic, pulmonic, portal, and renal. The systemic is the coursing of the arterial or oxygenated blood, propelled from the left side of the heart, through each and every part of the entire body, and the return current of venous blood, which is charged with the carbonic acid gas absorbed by the blood in the systemic circulation, to the

The Venæ Cavæ and Azygos Veins, with their Formative Branches.

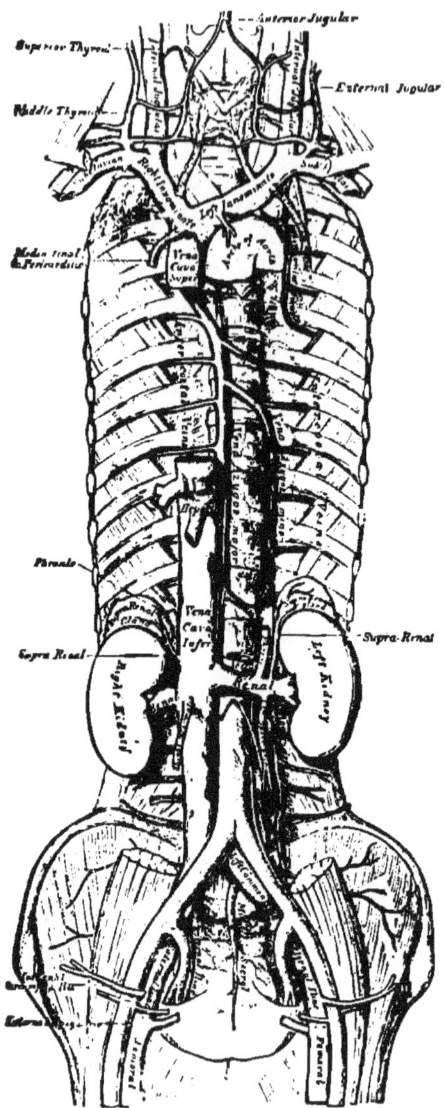

III.—View, from Front, of Main Blood-vessels leading to and from the Heart.

right side of the heart. The pulmonic comprises the coursing of the venous blood from the right side of the heart, outward, through the lungs, where it is purified, giving off the carbonic acid gas and absorbing fresh oxygen, and the return current of pure blood from the lungs to the left side of the heart. In the systemic circulation the arteries carry red blood, the veins purple; and the work of the capillaries is to exchange the elements which characterize the former for the latter. In the pulmonic, the arteries carry purple blood, the veins red, and the capillaries work an exchange of gases the reverse of that done in the systemic circulation.

Two distinct sounds accompany the heart's action. The contraction of the auricles forces the blood through the valves opening between the auricles and the ventricles, into the ventricles, which in turn contract, forcing the blood outward, the current from the right side into the pulmonary artery, and from the left side into the aorta. Three semilunar valves guard each of these openings from the heart, and prevent regurgitation of the blood into the heart when the ventricles are relaxed from the contraction. The first sound indicates the contraction of the walls of the heart, and impulse of the heart against the chest walls. The second is caused by the closing of the semilunar valves.

It may be interesting to trace the blood in its circuit through these two systems, and, for convenience, we will start at the left auricle, with the current freshly oxygenated from its circulation through the lungs.

The blood is forced through the valve opening between the left auricle and the left ventricle, into the left ventricle, and outward from the ventricle into the aorta, which gives off branches to the left and the right sides of the head, and to each arm; the large trunk continues downward in what is known as the abdominal aorta, giving off branches to internal organs, dividing at the pelvis, and extending down the legs. These are the main divisions, and they divide and subdivide, sending branches to every muscle, and these to every fibre of muscle, section of bone, skin, etc., the entire system being furnished with tiny arteries, the final subdivision of which is but one one-thousandth of an inch in diameter. These terminate in sections of capillaries.

The capillaries are interwoven like meshes

of lace-work, and the blood works its way through them, having no definite direction, but gradually approaching the tiny veins that draw the current from them. The veins join in a manner similar to the ramifications of the arteries, forming, finally, the main trunks, called the superior and inferior venæ cavæ, that receive the current from the members and organs, and dischauge it into the right auricle, to be forced, by the same contraction that takes place in the left auricle, through the orifice, into the right ventricle, and, by the contraction of the ventricles, out through the pulmonary arteries. Here the subdivisions are similar to those in the systemic circulation; the capillaries line the lung cells, and through their walls re-oxygenation takes place, which purifies the blood and renders it life-supporting again, the current passing on to the left side of the heart to continue its good work of body-building. The accompanying plate is a conventionalized plan of the systemic and pulmonic circulation. The light lines represent the arteries, and the dark, the venous currents.

The heart and the blood-vessels themselves do not derive their supply for rebuilding their own tissues from the blood they convey, but

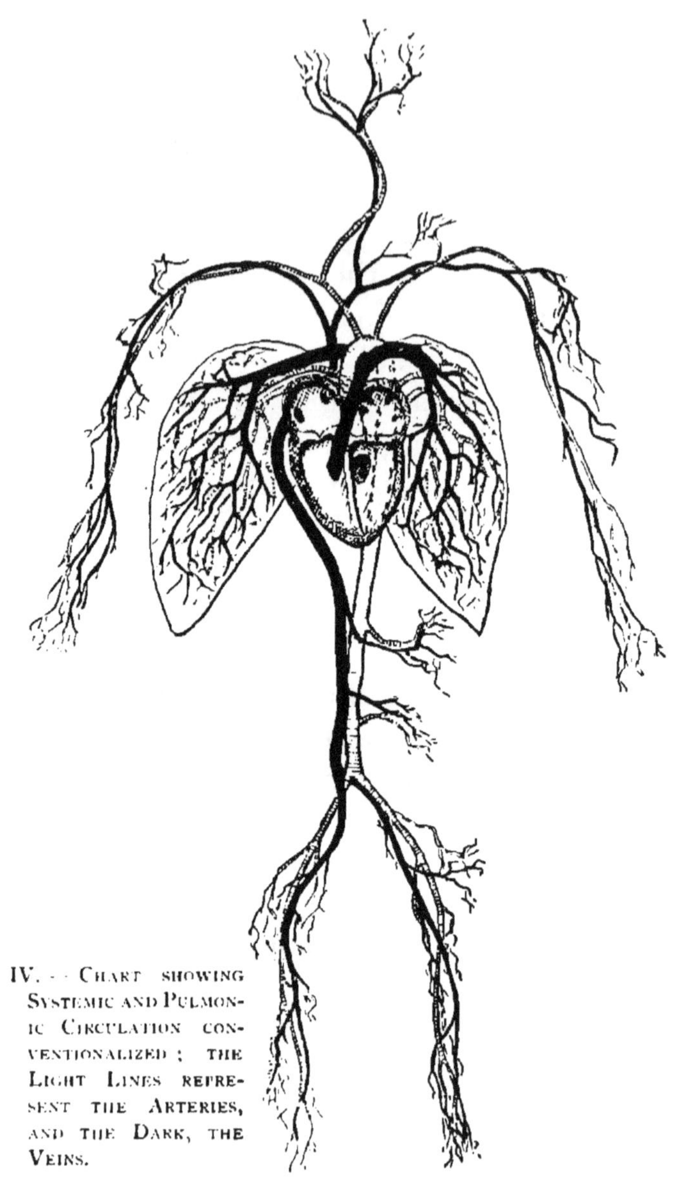

IV. — Chart showing Systemic and Pulmonic Circulation conventionalized; the Light Lines represent the Arteries, and the Dark, the Veins.

each is supplied with an independent system, which is a branch of the general system.

The portal circulation is for the absorption of nourishment from our foods. The abdominal aorta sends off large branches to the digestive apparatus, which invest the lining of the stomach and small intestine, and absorb, from the food matter, elements for body-building. The current continues on through the liver, where, in the capillaries, it gives off the material for making bile, and also undergoes chemical changes necessary to prepare it for its use in the systemic circulation. Continuing, it joins the inferior vena cava and mixes in the general current, to be forced through the pulmonic circulation, the last stage of preparation for its perfect work of tissue growth and repair.

The greater part of absorption takes place in the small intestine. The white of an egg, and other foods of this nature, however, are absorbed in the stomach, and relief from hunger by foods of this kind is marvellously quick. Rectal absorption also performs an important function in the sick-room, where artificial feeding is often a life-saving power. Absorption is more definitely described in the chapter on Digestion.

A drink of warm milk, or even water, will often allay hunger for a short period. The custom of sipping quite warm water an hour before meals is more than a fad. The stomach needs a bath, and the blood needs the liquid.

The renal circulation is a current less clearly understood by women than these other three, yet it holds a highly important place in the working of the human machine. A branch from the abdominal aorta passes through the kidneys, conveying a portion of the blood current. The subdivisions of this branch artery terminate in capillaries that invest the lining of the kidneys, whose function is to strain the water, with certain impurities, from the blood. It passes, in the form of urine, from the kidneys, through the ureters, into the bladder, and is thereafter expelled from that receptacle. The blood current, passing on, enters the inferior vena cava and mixes in the general circulation. The kidneys, and the preservation of their health, should be made a careful study. Physicians often find in the consumptive, the rheumatic, the gouty, traces of disease in the eliminations from these organs, long before the presence of such disease is noticeable else-

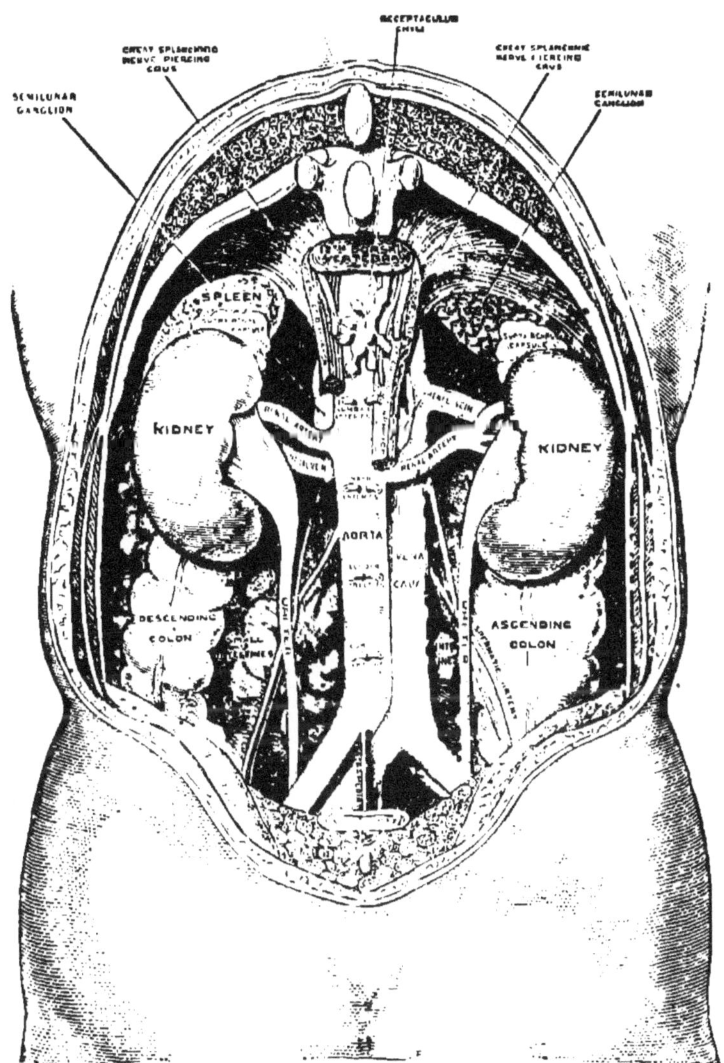

V.—SECTION OF BACK, SHOWING ORGANS OF RENAL CIRCULATION.

where. Physicians in treatment of renal obstructions often force profuse perspiration, and thus lighten the demands on these organs of elimination by aid of the pores of the skin. Nitrogenous refuse of food matter is largely eliminated through the kidneys, in form of urea, uric acid, and urates. Every one in this age of weak physical tendencies should watch carefully the tests these organs give of the development of health or disease. Kidneys, unlike lungs, seldom, if ever, give evidence of disease through suffering, hence the more need of watching signs.

Our aim in exercise should be to stimulate the capillary and venous circulation, and to improve the functions of all the organs. The daily occupations of life do not call for equal use of all our muscles, hence circulation is not equally active in all our tissues. In some instances, stiffness is the result, although loss of power is not especially noticeable. When circulation becomes sluggish, the impurities are not well eliminated, and disease threatens. If the blood reaching the tissues does not contain the elements to feed them, fatigue, and often pain, is certain to continue. The more rapid the circulation, the more completely the impurities of the blood are thrown off. This rapidity should not be overforced, however, and is best effected when the blood is amply supplied with oxygen and nourishment. Congestion is often due to lack of activity in capillaries and veins. This lack is often strongly marked in those past middle life.

Good circulation and good material for the body to utilize are of the greatest importance. If the heart action is vigorous, and the blood is forced continually to every part of the body, there is little opportunity for disease to develop, providing the digestive and respiratory apparatus do their work well. Arrested circulation causes, sooner or later, development of disease in whatever weak tissue we possess. It may result only in rendering us powerless to resist fatigue, colds, and congestion, or in the actual presence of defects, as gout, catarrh, rheumatism, etc.

Breathlessness, except from overexercise, is usually caused by some of the following reasons, viz.:

1. Lack of elasticity in chest walls or in lung tissue, rendering it impossible for the blood to become rapidly enough re-oxygenated to supply the demand.

2. Circulatory obstructions, as in portal and renal systems.

3. Cardiac weakness, due to weakness or disease of the heart muscles.

4. Alteration of valves by disease, permitting regurgitation of blood from heart's action.

5. Obesity, impeding heart's action.

The cause should always be ascertained, and discreet measures speedily adopted, else more unfavorable conditions will ensue.

In excess of exercise the heart labors in pumping the blood to overtaxed muscles for supplying the demand caused by rapid combustion, which has occasioned an excess of waste matter to be thrown into the blood, and which the blood cannot so rapidly eliminate. Oxygen cannot enter the blood until the carbonic acid gas is thrown off; the two phenomena work simultaneously.

Sometimes a lack of sufficient elasticity of lung tissue, or of the muscles which operate the lungs, is the cause of failure of these organs to purify the blood rapidly enough. In such the fault can be overcome by proper training. Sometimes, however, it is caused by lack of sufficient power in the heart itself. When this condition is present, violent exercise is extremely dangerous, and the point at which it should be stopped must be considered with great care by all athletes. This is not only necessary in case the heart is diseased or abnormal; overexertion will weaken the normal heart in every case. We may see this strongly emphasized in the "athlete's heart." It remains, therefore, for every person, whether athlete or otherwise, to find out what is overexertion in his case, and to stop short of that limit at all times. It may be a very low limit, and often is, especially in women; but, low or high, each should compare herself to herself, and not to her more vigorous neighbor.

CHAPTER V

RESPIRATION

"Seek the open air; the fruits which grow out doors are alone those which ripen in season."—BRINTON.

RESPIRATION is the term generally used to indicate the process by which the return blood current from the systemic circulation is purified in the lungs and rendered life-supporting again. The presence of carbonic acid in the blood, and the lack of and need of oxygen, cause the act of respiration. It is an imperative demand, one that we cannot resist voluntarily.

This act is performed mainly with the intercostal muscles, although chest, back, and abdominal muscles, as well as diaphragm and infracostals, aid in the process. Elasticity of lung tissue is also an essential in respiration. In enforced respiration, muscles known as the *serratus magnus* and *serratus posticus* (superior and inferior) and *scaleni* are principally employed.

In a complete respiration the chest is raised, the ribs somewhat straightened; *i. e.*, the articulation of the ribs with the vertebræ admits change of position, and the cartilaginous attachment against the "breast-bone" also yields, giving the ribs an appearance of extending more directly around the body than they do when in their normal position, which is a double curve; the intercostal spaces are widened, the diaphragm lowered, the cavity of the chest enlarged, and the lung cells opened. In order to make respiration complete, the arms should be raised; no other voluntary act, except forcing the intercostals, is advisable. Such directions as "lower the diaphragm," "breathe with the abdomen," etc., are unwise, and in some respects actually harmful, as the diaphragm and abdominal muscles should act secondarily only. The exhalation should immediately follow the inhalation, as the carbonic acid gas passes into the air of the lung cells as soon as the inspiration is made, and should be "breathed out." If held there, the blood, in its continuous circulation through the lungs, finds an insufficiency of oxygen in the partly exhausted air, and so passes on but poorly oxygenated. If there is necessarily any pause in respiration, let it be on the exhalation, not the inhalation.

The respiratory apparatus consists of larynx, pharynx, trachea, bronchi, and lungs. The nose should also have the dignity of being classed with these, since air is necessarily taken into the lungs through that organ. By exposure to the vascular mucous membrane of the narrow and winding nasal passages, the temperature of the air is normalized to meet the temperature of the body, and, to a certain extent, is purified before it enters the daintier structure of the lungs; foreign matter is lodged there, such as dust, etc., which would be injurious to lung tissue were it to be drawn within. During the inhalations the nostrils are expanded by special muscles, and the entrance of air facilitated. This action is noticeable in many people in normal breathing. It is especially so in enforced breathing, as with the horse after a hard drive. In some cases of paralysis these muscles are rendered useless, and nasal respiration is impaired. During the inspiration, the glottis is widely opened, and in the exhalation it is normalized. Thus, in unison with the rise and fall of the chest walls, and the widening and narrowing of the nostrils, we have the rhythmic opening and closing of the glottis.

The practice of breathing through the mouth is pernicious. It dries the saliva, thereby in-

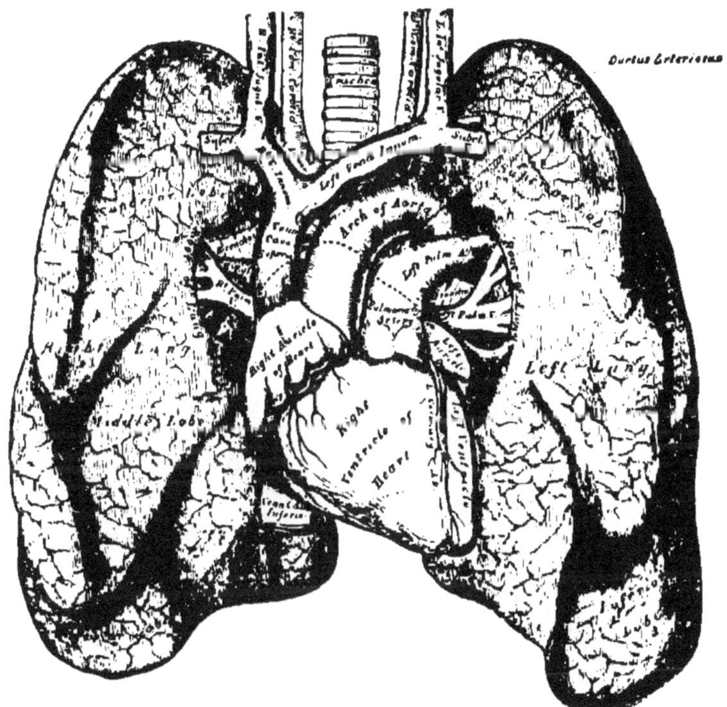

VI.—Organs of Pulmonic Circulation.

terfering with good digestion. The trachea also is dried, and catarrhal conditions of the throat and nose are the result.

The larynx and pharynx I will not describe.

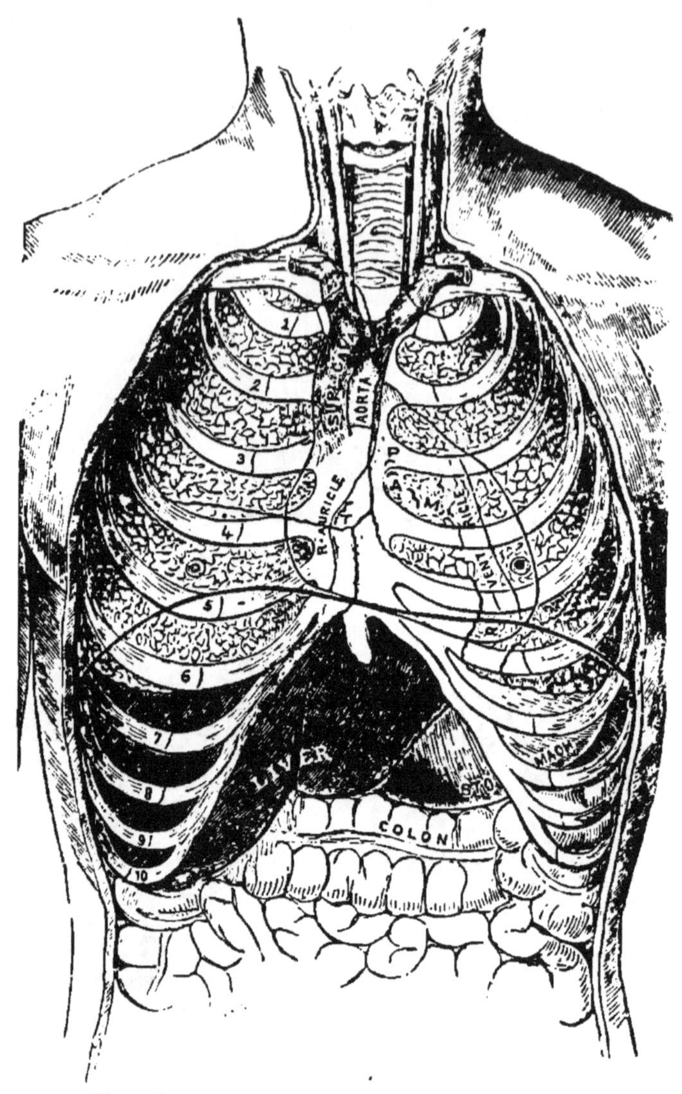

VII.—Lungs and Portion of Digestive Viscera.

Whenever any especial weakness of these is present, it should command the attention of a physician.

The trachea consists of a succession of carti-

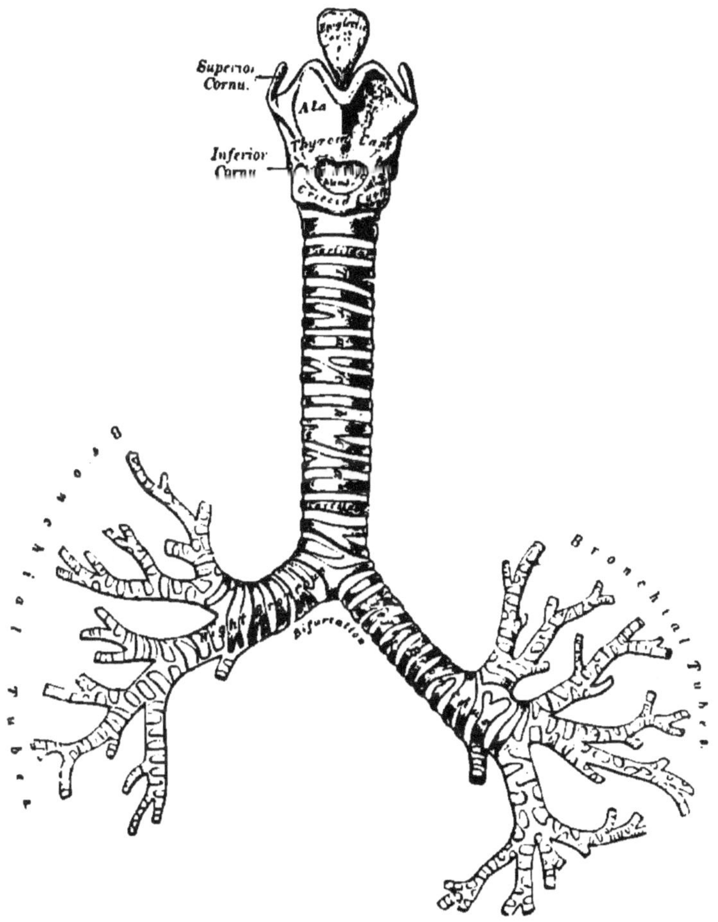

VIII.—Trachea and Bronchi.

laginous rings, connected by strong fibro-elastic tissue, forming a tube lined by a mucous membrane which is continuous throughout the respiratory apparatus.

In the chest this tube divides, sending a large branch to each lung—the one on the left dividing again into two branches, supplying the two lobes which constitute the left lung; and the right, into three branches, supplying the three lobes which constitute the right lung.

These main branches divide and infinitely subdivide, growing more delicate in structure at each subdivision, until finally the cartilaginous rings disappear, and only the thin mucous lining, on a base of elastic fibrous tissue, remains. These are known as the "ultimate bronchial tubes," and are about one twenty-fifth of an inch in diameter. Each dainty "ultimate bronchial tube" terminates in a division of lung about one-twelfth of an inch in diameter, called a lobule. This encloses a cavity which is divided into scores of tiny cells, or vesicles, about one two-hundredth to one seventy-fifth of an inch in diameter. Each vesicle is covered on its exterior with a lacework of capillary blood-vessels, and the walls of these blood-vessels admit the exchange of gases, the phenomenon which, in addition to the work done in the systemic capillaries, is called respiration. In the pulmonary capillaries the impure carbonic acid gas is thrown off from the blood, and pure oxygen takes its place; in the systemic, the oxygen is absorbed into the tissues, and carbonic acid gas takes its place.

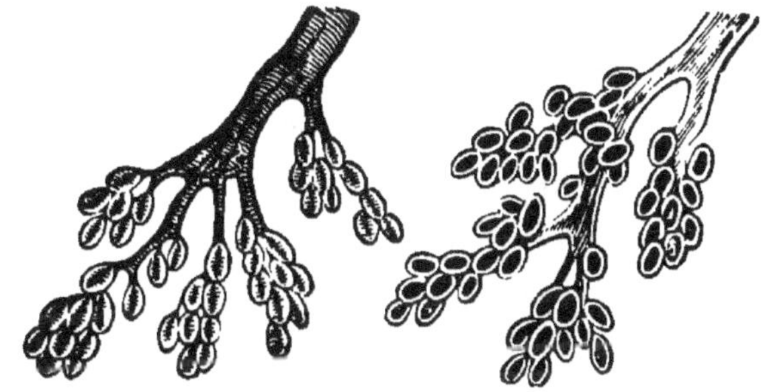

IX.—Terminal Bronchial Tubes and Lobules.

The chemical change is identical with the process of combustion. Body fuel is consumed in the great human furnace, and the refuse removed by the blood, and, to a great extent, eliminated by the lungs; although skin and kidneys are equally valuable sewers in the work allotted them by nature.

The more flexible the lungs, the more surface is exposed for action of air, and the better oxygenated will the blood be. It is impossible to calculate the extent of surface presented in a pair of elastic lungs. Scherling estimates it at fifteen hundred square feet, so great is the multiplicity of the minute vesicles, and the elasticity of the partitions between them.

The temperature of the air inhaled changes during respiration. The longer it is retained, the nearer it approaches the temperature of the body. This varies more with deep than with light breathing. Air loses somewhat in quantity in the process of respiration, due to the fact that oxygen is used in some parts of the body; it also loses about four per cent. oxygen and gains four per cent. carbonic acid gas in the lungs. It also gains ammonia, organic matter, and other impurities, which, to a certain extent, occasion the bad odors of breath ; although catarrh, disease of teeth or throat, and unhealthy conditions of stomach and other digestive organs, are largely responsible for them.

This shows the great importance of living in and constantly breathing pure, clean air. Lungs are doorways to good health. While kidneys and skin do valuable work in eliminating impurities of the body, no other organs can do the work the lungs have to do in reoxygenation of the blood. It is especially important that they be evenly clad—not overheated by air-tight clothing for the lower chest, and chilled by insufficient clothing for the upper; not restricted by tight clothing, nor depressed by bad posture. If cramped by posture and clothing, they can expose but a comparatively small portion of their surface to air, and the work of reoxygenation is incomplete. It is of the utmost importance that our living-rooms should be well ventilated. Office, boudoir, and school-room should have a constant current of air circulating through them. Every exhalation carries with it a certain amount of vapors and of waste organic and animal matter, the refuse of the body; and if we breathe into the lungs this once-breathed air, we absorb into our blood the refuse of our own or of others' bodies. The organic matter exhaled through the lungs is so actively poisonous that an accumulation of it injected into the blood of a rabbit will produce death.

Many people who would revolt at the idea of eating mouldy bread, sour vegetables, or tainted meat, do not hesitate to sit in crowded, poorly-ventilated rooms, and poison their blood by inhaling impurities; by such abuse they are rendered susceptible to colds and to disease which they would be able to resist were their blood properly oxygenated by breathing pure air.

It is poor economy to consider that fuel is wasted unless rooms are air-tight, so that every atom of heat is utilized. Ventilate properly, dress comfortably, and heat apartments sufficiently for comfort.

Chilling sensations, even for other parts of the body than the chest, are liable to react on the throat and lungs. Congestion in the tissues of the throat produces hoarseness or irritation. Massage, described in the chapter on Massage, if carefully applied while these ills are in their incipiency, will help greatly in allaying suffering. Congestion is much more serious when it takes the form of " bronchial weakness," as it is often called, extending into the chest, and interfering with the free passage of air to the lung cells. Congestion of the lungs is another grave condition of weak tissues. In this the entire respiratory tract becomes involved, and it is serious in proportion to extent of congestion, condition of patient, etc. This, with congestion in the current that supplies the lung cells with tissue-building material, constitutes the first stage of pneumonia. I mention these facts to urge attention to errors in their incipiency. Too many neglect sending for the physician until severe suffering is present, and then it is often too late for him to prescribe successfully for the patient's recovery.

CHAPTER VI

DIGESTION

"Now good digestion wait on appetite, and health on both."—SHAKSPEARE.

A TORPID liver causes a morbid mind, and an acid stomach, acidity of temper.

The question, "Is life worth living?" has been facetiously answered: "It depends on the liver."

On health of digestive apparatus, health of body largely depends. Were the blood always supplied with elements necessary for rebuilding the tissues of the body, including, of course, oxygen, as well as food material, the lack of vital health would be comparatively small. The blood, if starved for want of good material for body-building, can do but little good work, and pain and exhaustion are sure to follow sooner or later.

The cases are rare where loss of strength comes from an insufficient quantity of food. The lack is from foods not being properly utilized, and this lack of economy in nature is due to some of the following reasons:

1. Indiscriminate selection of food material.

2. Improper preparation of same.

3. Lack of cheer and of wholesome table topics.

4. Nervous, hurried mastication, and other pernicious habits.

5. Weak condition of some portion of digestive apparatus.

6. Foods taken in too large quantities. We loathe the individual who confesses he has "eaten too much."

7. Too long intervals from meal to meal, or the habitual eating "between meals," except in cases of invalidism, when frequent feeding is necessary.

In this chapter I shall deal mainly with the fifth.

Of the first two I will say that research in regard to proportion of food ingredients for nourishing the human animal is claiming the attention of scientists, but that opinions differ so widely that each individual must still discriminate largely for himself. The influences of different foods on different diseases can now be studied, as we have able authority on these subjects; and by making one's heredity and environment also a study, the selection of foods need not be entirely experimental.

Generally we rear our thoroughbred animals more scientifically than we do our children. Their foods are known to be hygienic and well apportioned. Through generations of research, our physicians have gained a knowledge of the influence of drugs on health and disease, while little actual labor has been expended on testing the internal laboratory in its ability to adapt the different food elements for good or for harm in the various conditions of health and disease existing there, and diet has, in consequence, been largely experimental.

Individuals, however, differ so widely in physical conditions, in tendencies to disease, and in temperament, that individual study will always be necessary, even under the best of scientific research. Climatic influence, conditions of nervousness and of fatigue, amount of physical and mental labor to be performed, also enter strongly into consideration in the selection of foods. Very few find their daily requirements can be met by duplicating the preceding day's *régime*.

The rational thinker, if he possesses good

digestive organs, can safely allow his appetite to be his dietetic adviser. It has been proved in the training of athletes that the truly healthy appetite craves only wholesome foods. The craving for pickles, spices, and sweets is abnormal, and should not be indulged.

Let articles of diet be judiciously selected, properly cooked, and prudently eaten, and nature may then be relied upon to do her work thoroughly, if digestive organs are healthy, and lungs are plentifully supplied with fresh air.

Of old the palate ran riot, regardless of unhygienic results. The cook was lauded for her savory dishes and pastries. Each hostess vied with her neighbor in table attractions, and a meal of simple, healthful foods was almost unknown. Gastronomical debaucheries were in vogue, and still these good dames preached temperance; and we descendants of these estimable women continue our intemperate eating, and continue to preach temperance. Consistency is indeed a jewel rare. Let us preach temperance, but let us understand the full definition of the term, and practice it in eating, as in drinking. "Cocktails and caramels" are physiologically synonymous in their results.

Let us eat to live, not live to eat; remembering that the delicacies that tickle the palate for the moment, may conspire to wreck the home by inducing invalidism.

One cannot be too particular that influences at meals shall be of a wholesome and agreeable nature. Be good friends with the foods that are to nourish the body, and avoid unfavorable comment on them. Select from what is provided, but do not pamper an abnormal desire for any one article of food.

Brinton, in his "Pursuit of Happiness," says of our living-rooms, that they should be "light, dry, bright, and airy; well ventilated, equably warmed, appropriately furnished; free from bad odors, far from brutal noises, screened from impertinent curiosity." This should be emphatically observed in our dining-rooms. We digest with our food the mental influences with which we surround ourselves; and these influences follow us, not only while that especial meal is nourishing our bodies, but through life; as no one day can be isolated in its influences from life entire. Contrast the individual who eats moderately, both as to quantity and speed, with the nervous, hurried eater, and you will see a similar contrast in endurance, health, nerve force, and consequent usefulness. Disease and human suffering should never be permitted as table topics. Discuss, instead, health, and immunity from such ills. The daily papers should only be opened at pages that breathe peace and good will to all; not disease and peril.

The disciplining of children should not be carried on at table, and finance and scandal should also be tabooed.

We will assume that the foods are wisely selected and properly prepared, and discuss the more practical side of the subject, health of the digestive organs. The digestive apparatus consists of mouth, esophagus, stomach, pancreas, liver, duodenum, small intestine, and colon. Each part has its individual work to perform in the great internal laboratory, and each will do that work if properly treated. These hidden organs work with wonderful intelligence. If any neglect happens, discord is sure to follow.

Foods are classified as organic and inorganic. The inorganic include salts, mixed with other foods, and water, used either alone or with other foods. Fully four glasses of water per day should be drunk, but not with food. It is best also to drink sterilized water only. For the home let it be boiled, cooled, bottled, and put on ice. Ice should not be used in the

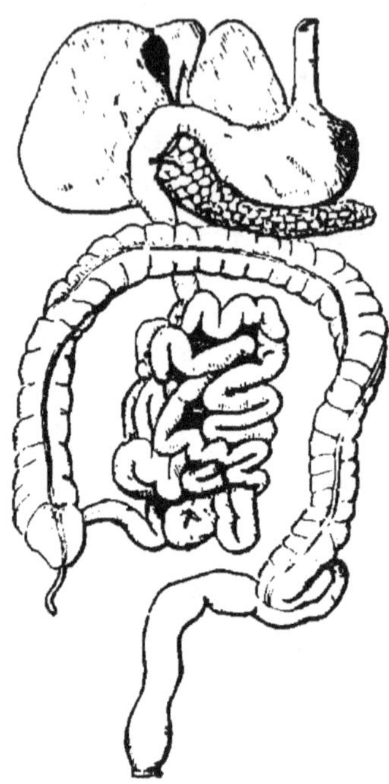

X.—Digestive Apparatus, showing Liver, Bile Duct, Stomach, Pancreas, Duodenum, Small Intestine, and Colon.

water, even though sterilized ice is used. It chills the stomach and impairs the health.

The organic foods comprise the nitrogenous, or tissue-building, and the non-nitrogenous, or fuel-foods. The former include albuminoids from the animal, and gluten and legumen from the vegetable, kingdom ; and the latter, fats and carbo-hydrates. The body to be well nourished and supplied with good material for usefulness needs a proportionate amount of both, and these should be varied from day to day. An excess of either will overtax some of the digestive organs, and a lack of either causes impoverishment in some of the tissues.

It is generally conceded that meat diet is taken in excess in this country, especially by children and nervous people. Butter, olive oil, and cream are good substitutes for it.

Bread or cereals, vegetables, milk, and fruits ripened naturally, not forced, should form part of every meal, but neither should predominate. Meats are not necessary with these, except where especial strength is required.

It is best that sharp-seed fruits and berries be stewed and strained before they are eaten. Strawberries, tomatoes, and pineapples are not considered prudent diet for those of rheumatic tendency.

Starchy foods and sweets should be avoided by those inclined to obesity.

Only natural acids, such as lemon juice,

should be used on the table; vinegar should be avoided.

Excess in potato diet is unwise.

Whole wheat flour should be substituted for fine flour.

We need more fuel foods in winter than in summer.

In the matter of sweets and condiments there is much intemperate indulgence.

Food matter is converted into a liquid before the blood absorbs it. This phenomenon is accomplished in the digestive laboratory through heat, motion, and natural juices which are supplied through the glands of these organs.

Digestion begins in the mouth by the food matter mixing with saliva. By this process, starch is converted into sugar. Good teeth, slow mastication, and an avoidance of artificial liquids while chewing the food are requisites for this degree of digestion. Gladstone, that marvel of self-preservation, has thirty-two incisions as his standard for chewing; or, more clearly speaking, he chews thirty-two times each mouthful of food. As much as this is necessary. Bread should always be eaten with cereals so as to make mastication a necessity, otherwise the cereal is very apt to be swallowed without a sufficient amount of saliva, and the first stage of digestion is consequently incomplete.

The food is swallowed, and passes down the esophagus and into the stomach. Here it undergoes another process of digestion through the involuntary action of the stomach walls, called the peristaltic motion, which twists and churns the food matter, mixing it with the gastric juices that are given off through the glands of the stomach lining. The mass thus prepared is called chyme.

Nitrogenous foods are mainly digested and absorbed in the stomach; and while the non-nitrogenous undergo a chemical change there, other elements are required in their complete preparation. These elements are the bile and the pancreatic juice. These mix with the food matter on its passage out from the stomach through the duodenum. They not only digest the non-nitrogenous food, but they also convert starch, the digestion of which was begun in the mouth, into soluble sugar.

From fifteen to thirty minutes are required to prepare the chyme for absorption. Stomach digestion, even of our heartiest meal, should be completed in from four to five hours; if it remains in the stomach longer than that,

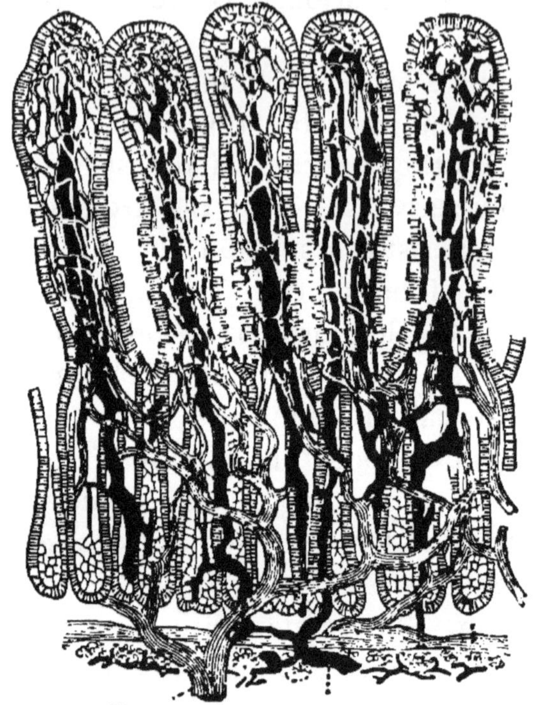

XI.—INTESTINAL VILLI MAGNIFIED FROM ONE-EIGHTIETH OF AN INCH.

the matter becomes putrid, and unfit for absorption.

The more complete process of absorption takes place in the small intestine. This measures about twenty feet (approximate) in an adult, and constitutes the greater portion of the digestive tract. It is lined with a membrane of tiny little organs of velvety appearance, called intestinal villi. These are like intelligent little tongues, and suck in the food properties through their walls. The liquid made from the digested matter is called chyle, and is absorbed by means of lymphatics into the blood in the portal circulation. The food is propelled through the intestine by the vermicular force, and the same force propels the undigested portions, with other refuse food matter, into the colon, and thence out of the body. The passage of food through the alimentary canal covers about twelve hours in the healthy adult.

The digestive apparatus should be carefully guarded from harm. If perfect health exists there, consciousness of digestion, or of a stomach, will never be experienced.

The stomach requires space for work, and compression from tight or stiff clothing is sure to result in unhealthy conditions.

Indigestion is not always recognized, except in acute forms of stomach weakness. There are other, graver conditions that work havoc with good health and endurance. Fatigue, suscep-

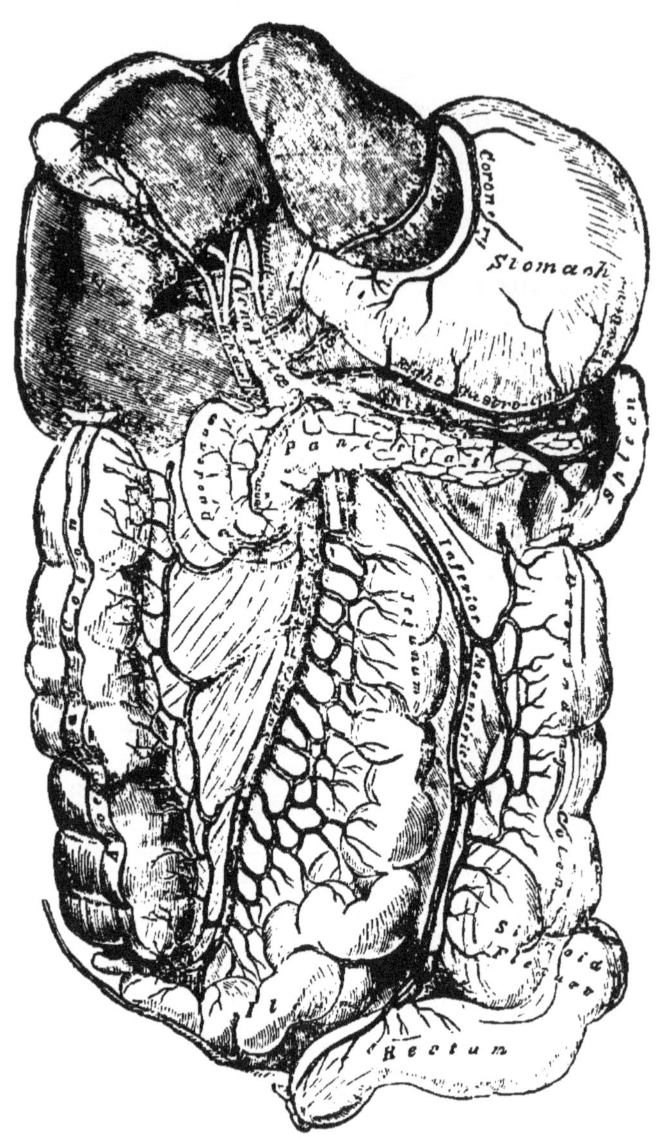

XII.—The Great Portal Circulation.

tibility to colds, to cold, to disease, are apt to have their origin in weakness of some of the digestive organs. If the food element is not well prepared in each and every section of the digestive tract, lack of assimilation is sure to follow, and pain and fatigue are the result. The child or adult is fortunate when nature gives warning in form of acute conditions, as then greater care is used in choice of foods. A careful selection of nourishing foods, a cup of hot water sipped an hour before meals, and the practice of well-arranged exercise to improve the functions of the digestive apparatus, are items of much advantage. Neither mental nor physical exertion should immediately follow a hearty meal. When excessive physical fatigue is present, foods of easily digestible quality must be chosen. Tired nerves of internal organs, as of organs of locomotion, should never be taxed.

Normal hunger is the cry of the blood for food, and to obtain it the blood is called in large quantities to the digestive apparatus, where it should be allowed to remain until the process of stomach digestion is completed. When too hurried to allow proper time for mastication and digestion, it is best to take no

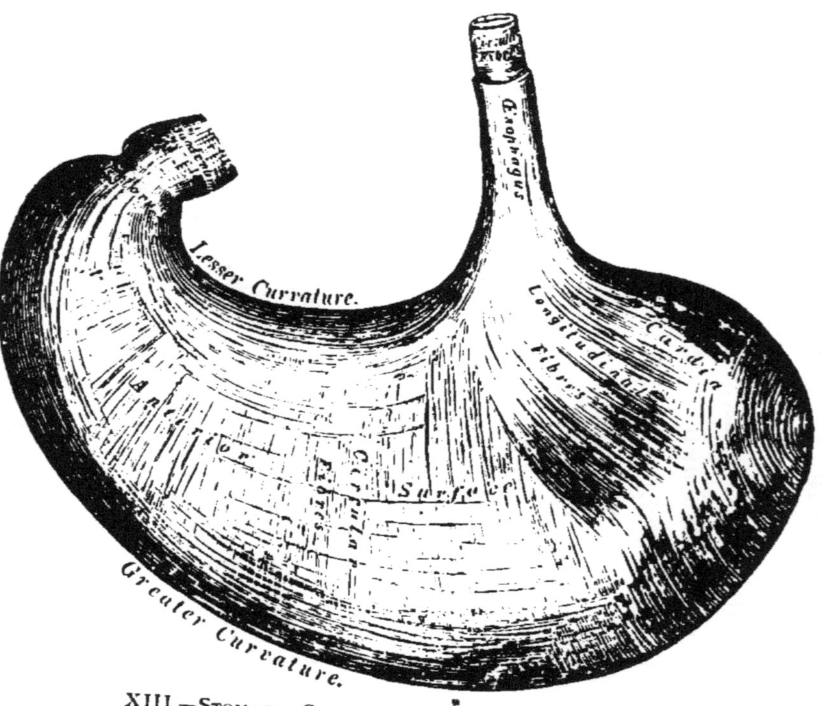

XIII.—Stomach, Showing Outer Muscular Coat.

food other than some warm liquid diet. The schoolboy who rushes home to luncheon, gulps meat and other solids, and rushes out either to sports or to resume his studies, lays a foundation for weak conditions that will at least render him incapable of resisting fatigue, colds, and disease, even if acute indigestion does not follow. In order to establish good digestive conditions, a child should be required to sit a proper length of time at the table, to insure against hurried eating.

Candy-eating and gum-chewing waste the juices of the mouth and stomach by keeping them active to no purpose. I have heard that some physicians recommend gum-chewing to their dyspeptic patients. It is probably the only possible way of causing them to introduce saliva into their too-hurriedly masticated food-matter. Were they to chew their foods properly, they would not need the gum.

Hunger should not be allowed to continue. A slice of well-buttered bread, an egg (beaten with milk, if desired), a cup of clam broth, matzoon, warm milk, bouillon, some easily-digested fruit, or even a cup of hot water, will prove a valuable between-meal luncheon, and should be an established habit with people of light digestive power, or when light meals are found to be necessary. Delicate people and invalids had best habituate themselves to frequent light meals, rather than attempt to force their stomachs to handle more material.

A person should not retire hungry; some plan of light nourishment, as described in the foregoing paragraph, should be observed.

The heartiest meal had best be made at evening, when the cares of the day are over, and digestion is liable to be uninterrupted by mental or physical labor.

These three apparatuses—circulatory, respiratory, and digestive—may well be called the trinity of existence. If either be out of repair, the others are crippled. The circulatory can do but little work for the body if the respiratory does not keep the blood well supplied with oxygen, and if the digestive does not properly prepare the food matter for absorption. The digestive needs equally good co-labor from the circulatory and the respiratory, and the respiratory from the other two. Hence the title, tripod of existence, may be aptly applied to these three, for they form the support of the element called life.

The question naturally arises, " What shall I

do to inherit eternal life?" For that is what health to the end of our days should mean. The solution is, first study well the conditions of the digestive organs, and make fresh air and systematized exercise a daily care. The lessons in this book are especially arranged to improve and preserve the health of these organs.

CHAPTER VII

CONCERNING THE SPINE

"As the twig is bent, the tree is inclined."

A WEAK spine causes weak execution of strong ambitions.

Posture involves a study of the mechanical as well as of the physiological laws of our bodies.

Mechanically, the trunk is a cylinder, and the spine is the supporting shaft on which all the parts are suspended. The spine, or spinal column as it should be called, consists of a number of irregular bones (twenty-four) called vertebræ. These are freely movable upon one another, and are separated by disks of cartilage which serve to protect the spine, and consequently the brain, from jar. The spinal column is so formed that it encloses a canal which contains the spinal cord, or nerve matter which is transmitted from the brain, and given off in branches at every vertebra into opposite pairs of nerves. These, with their various subdivisions, help to make up the nervous system.

The spinal muscular system consists of five layers, sixty muscles in all. Lack of space in this volume prevents detailed explanation. I will simply say, in brief, that these not only band the spine together and control each part of it, but connect with it every member of the body and control every movement. Not a breath is drawn, not a finger stirred, but the spine feels its influence.

In the infant the spine is straight; but when walking begins, the four normal curves which characterize the adult spine (shown in cut XIV.) gradually appear. These aid mechanically in the poise of the body, and physiologically in preventing jar to the brain from heavy walking on heels, jumping, or other shock.

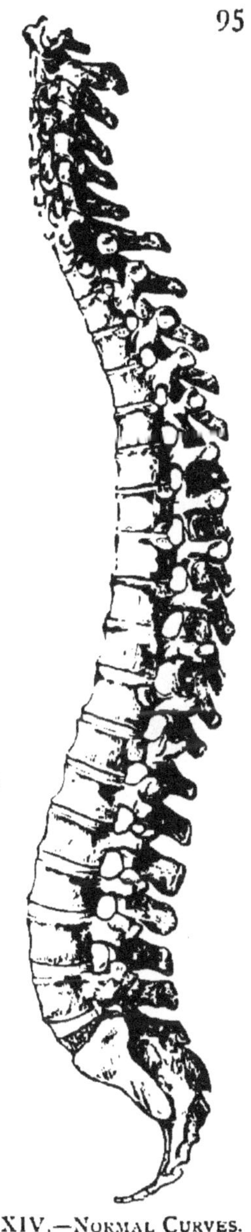

XIV.—NORMAL CURVES.

The spine supports the head, arms, chest, and pelvis; and is supported by, and transmits the supported weight to, the lower limbs. The weight should rest equally upon both legs, so that the muscles on either side of the spine will be used with equal tension, and the normal position be maintained.

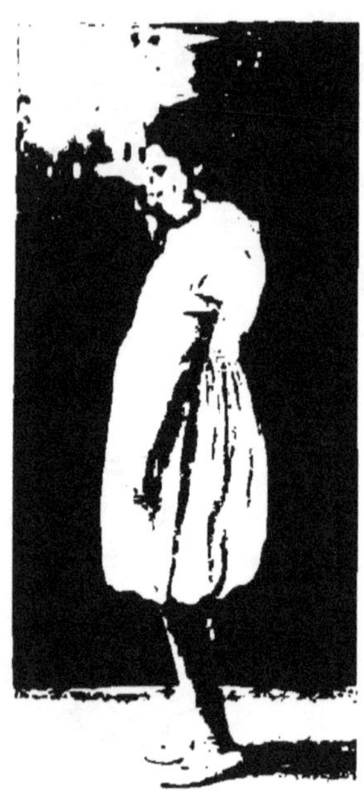

XV. Careless Standing Posture. Habitual with Many Children.

The head is supported in an upright position by certain muscles attached to the upper portion of the spine, and should not be allowed to droop forward; neither should the weight of the arms be suspended from the front of the body; in either case, as a result, the chest droops, and the four normal curves of the spine become exaggerated. The request, "Throw back your shoulders," is more than useless, as such an attempt would cause still further protrusion forward of the abdomen, and a still more depressed condition of the chest. The direction, "Raise the chest," is more rational, but even this should be explained. Simultaneously with the raising of the chest, the hips should be drawn back, so that the pelvis is supported at its proper angle, and the pelvic organs thereby are maintained in their natural position. To be accurate in poise of body, the pubic arch (the angle formed by the union of the two bones at the front and lower part of the trunk) should be fully half an inch back of the clavicular notch (the union of the collar-bones).

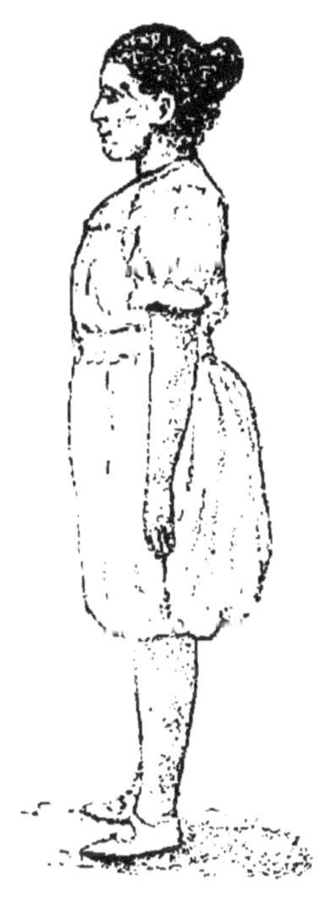

XVI.—Accurate Standing Posture.

More easily, perhaps, can we obtain the correct posture by keeping the chest and the abdomen in vertical line.

The legs form an arch for the support of the body, and the foot an arch for the support of each leg, heel and toe together doing their work. The weight of the body should stand directly over the thigh and leg bones, which are directly over the arch of the foot, the calf and thigh muscles being tense. The two feet should be at an angle of ninety degrees, whether the heels are in touch or otherwise. This angle forms a base that corresponds to the poise of the weight of the body in its suspension from the spine, and is necessary in order to economize strength and to attain repose while standing. Lax knee muscles always indicate a laxity or lack of vigor in spinal muscles.

Lateral curvature is a deviation of the spine to the right or left from its normal position. It often results from an unequal use of the spinal muscles, causing preponderance of strength on the one side and a lax condition of the muscles on the opposite side. The intervertebral disks are capable of slight compression, and from long-continued, unequal pressure brought to bear upon the concave side, they become a trifle narrower on that than on the convex side. It is not considered that this condition is permanent in incipient cases, but that it normalizes itself during the hours of rest. Deviation from the normal spine can be easily detected by the mother, and should receive prompt attention. It may be due to natural conditions, such as hereditary weakness, malnutrition, sleeping in poorly-ventilated rooms, or other influences which lower the stamina. Or it may be the result of mechanical causes, such as uneven heels, clothing that binds or drags, standing with weight unequally supported, carrying parcels (schoolbooks, for instance), and other means which overtax the muscles on one side, while the corresponding ones on the opposite side are comparatively in disuse. This inequality is emphasized by gravitation, until the child begins unconsciously to maintain this posture, even in his sleep. The only remedy is to remove the cause, and use rational gymnastic exercise for the restoration of the disused muscles and for normalizing the poise. I will describe three tests that the mother can easily apply for detecting deviation of spine. These tests should be made at least once in every three months with growing children.

1. Undress the child, and then, without admonishing him to "straighten up," allow him to assume his natural posture. With the fingers trace the spine down its entire length, beginning at the first prominent vertebra, at the base of the neck. Mark successively each ver-

tebra, or a sufficient number to show the exact line of the spine, with dots of ink applied with a small brush. Then mark a straight line down the back, or use a plumb-line, and note the deviation from the perpendicular. For further memoranda, place rulers under the arm-pits, allowing them to rest on the hips, and note whether or not the space at the waist line is equal at both sides. Another test is to alternate the weight of the trunk from one foot to the other, and observe whether or not the waist presents an equal depth of hollow on each side. Also note the position of the shoulder-blades in their relation to the spine. They should be evenly adjusted, and firm against the other tissues, not protruding like wings.

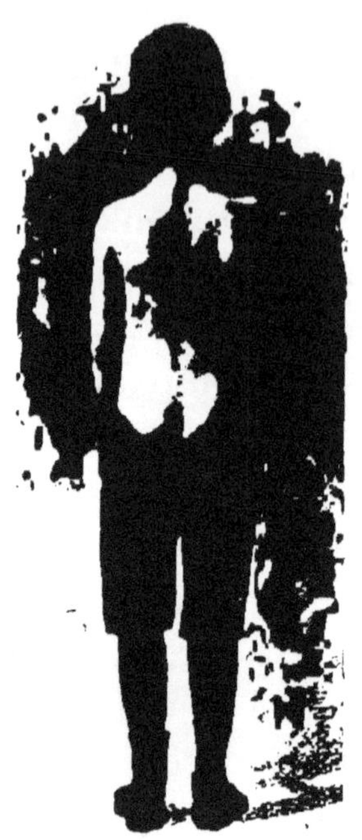

XVII.—Test with Ink-spots for Spinal Deviation.

2. Request the child to stand erect. Tie a soft cord loosely around the neck, holding the

knot at the prominent bone before mentioned, at the base of the neck. (Cut XVIII.) Request the child to bend his body slowly forward. (Cut XIX.) Repeat four or five times. If the spine line, indicated by the ink-dots, falls away from the plumb-line repeatedly in the same direction, that divergence indicates the curvature as regards lateral deviation; but if it rests on alternate sides, or directly on the column, it is probable that no curvature is present.

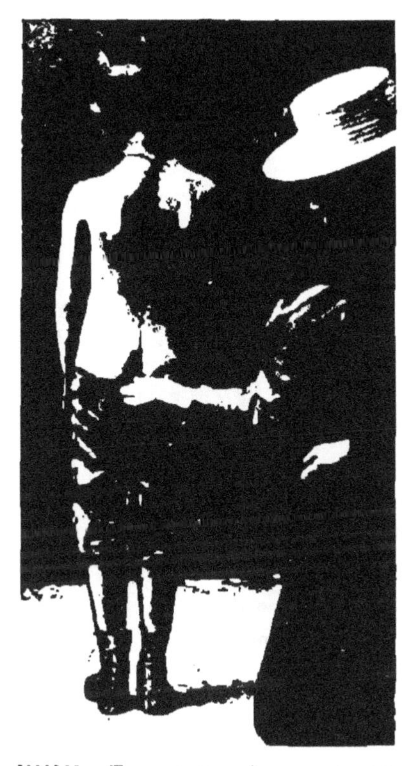

XVIII.—Test with Ink-spots and Plumb-line for Spinal Deviation.

3. Request the child to stand erect, with closed eyes, and to raise his arms slowly to the height of the shoulders; then note whether or not one arm is below the plane of the other.

This helps to determine the condition of the spine.

These simple tests are easily applied, and may be implicitly relied on. When they show irregularity of strength, or loss of intermediate position of spinal muscles, that is, when those on one side show preponderance of strength over those on the other, medical advice should be sought.

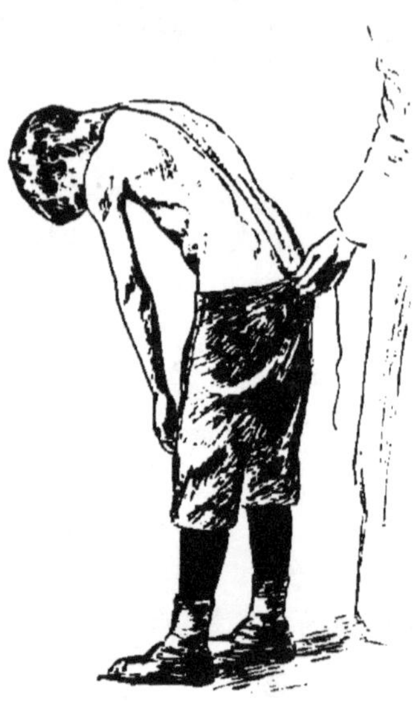

XIX.—Test Described in II Showing Trunk Bend.

I have referred only to simple or single curvature. Compound curvature, or cases that are already in the hands of the specialist, need no mention here. This volume is only for home tests, and for study of defects in their incipiency.

Irregularities of the spine often begin in early babyhood, from improper handling, etc. This subject is treated more at length in the chapter on Early Life and Training of Children.

The sitting posture, both at home and at school, also requires careful consideration. Many children are allowed to sit at desks and tables too high for them, while others are provided with those too low; the encouragement to irregular posture in either case is inevitable. Let this be avoided, even though it incurs expense and trouble. The object is to properly rear a human being, and we should not dare jeopardize his health and future interests by allowing unhygienic influences to destroy them. A very common error, and one that scarcely ever occurs to the parent as such, is the custom of allowing children to sit habitually in chairs too deep for them. The chair seat should measure the same length as

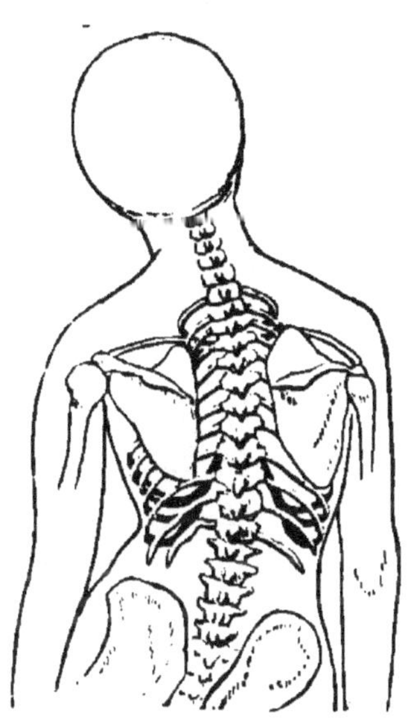

XX.—Position of Spine in Simple (Right) Lateral Curvature.

(Arranged by Dr. Mosher.)

the child from under the bent knee to the back. In this way a suitable support for the upper spine is given by resting the lower spine firmly against the back of the chair, thereby establishing the point of leverage at the lower spine, instead of at the waist, as is the case in careless posture. Then, if the mother requests the child to crowd far back on his chair, the mechanical law of leverage will tend to prevent any drooping forward of the spine. Change this point of leverage, and we get the deformity so common among boys—the deformity that is wrecking the health and manly carriage of many male bicycle riders. Let us hope that pride may come to their rescue before the next generation of men are hopelessly deformed.

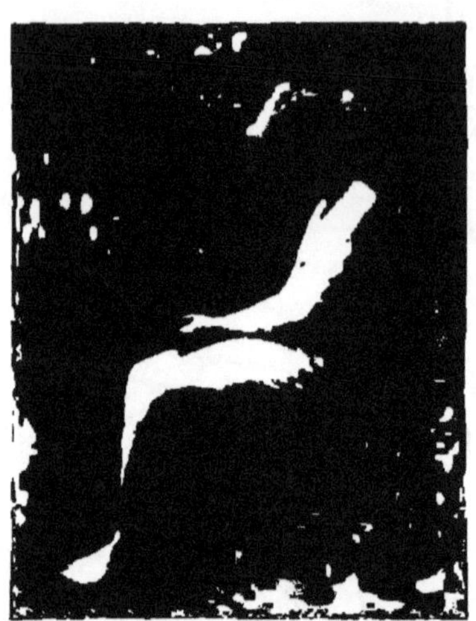

XXI. Careless Sitting Posture, Habitual with Some.

Sitting month after month in a schoolroom,

with the light coming continually from one and the same side; one-sided games, like croquet; wearing of high heels, which causes an unnatural position of the spine at the waist line; narrow-toe shoes, causing the weight of the body to be supported too much on the heels; corset pressure, causing the pelvis to tilt forward; heavy skirts, dragging at the back and causing the spine to assume a straight line from the waist down, and consequently throwing the abdomen forward, all have a deplorable effect on spinal muscles, and consequently upon the nerves and internal organs. In some cases of incorrect posture, many of the muscles would, nevertheless, work correctly were the mechanical interferences referred to removed; but, un-

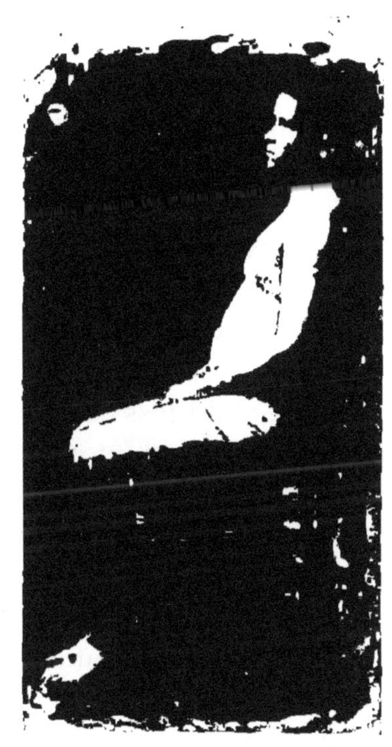

XXII.—Accurate Sitting Posture.

fortunately, they are allowed to remain, and their baleful influence increases slowly, day by day; so slowly that in many cases actual deformity is present before the mother is aware of it.

Had she but known how to detect it in its incipiency, and then employed proper means for counteracting it, it would never have established itself. It is unfortunate when the mother, through neglect or ignorance, passes over slight defects as meaningless, or as something the child will outgrow, or as the "fate of humanity generally." For even if actual deformity does not result, defects of any nature make the child less able to resist colds, fatigue, and the development of inherited tendencies to disease; while the mere consciousness of physical imperfection has often a baleful effect upon the mind of the possessor, of itself sufficient argument for endeavoring earnestly to overcome all unfavorable influences for the child.

Perfection of form, grace of carriage, repose of manner, and ease of posture, have far more than mere beauty of feature to do with realizing the highest type of female loveliness.

I will close this chapter with a quotation from one of my lectures that has been copied in many public prints throughout the country:

"The natural posture of the American girl is by no means graceful. No matter how pretty a face may be, its beauty is entirely lost unless it is poised over a figure that is natural, graceful, and dignified. Careless posture gives rise, sooner or later, to careless traits in character, if, indeed, they do not already exist."

CHAPTER VIII

SWEDISH EXERCISES FOR THE HOME

"Le physique gouverne toujours le morale."—VOLTAIRE.

GYMNASTIC movements are often too heavy to bring about absolute harmony of health. People are apt to consider that light movements are childish, and of their own preference they undertake those of too fatiguing a nature, with consequent disadvantage. The aim in physical training is to acquire health and skill, and with this end in view, we must employ a system of work that is based on strength of the vital organs, and that, in consequence, will not overtax them. While muscular development and reduction of adipose are important, the internal organs, especially the heart and lungs, must not be overtaxed in their attainment. Coördination of will power and muscle, flexibility, skill—these, not muscular power, should be the first attainments. The condition of unused muscles, and the relation of strength between these and the over-used ones, must also receive attention in the arrangement of work, both in amount and variety, else symmetry cannot be established and maintained. These are accessories to organic health, which is our highest purpose. For such work, the Swedish system of gymnastics offers the best advantages.

It is simple, safe, and scientific, easily learned, and readily applied.

Dr. Benjamin Lee, in Hare's "Practical Therapeutics," says of it, "Movement, or motion, is in modern philosophy the initial of every physical phenomenon or process. Heat, light, electricity, the attractions, are all 'modes of motion,' to use the generally adopted phrase. In these instances, however, the demonstration of motion is often difficult, sometimes impossible. When we come to the consideration of the living animal, however, the phenomena and processes which we call vital, this difficulty vanishes. In the primordial cell of every living tissue we are able, with the aid of a microscope, to see this motion going on. This cell is the unit and exponent of life, both in its origin and its perpetuation. We observe the incessant movement of its contents within and through its walls by constant endosmose and exosmose. Irregularity or retardation of this motion constitutes the condition to which we give the name 'disease.' Cessation of this motion is 'death.' 'Health,' is that condition of the individual in which the movements of the cell contents of all the tissues are normally carried on. It is the function of ordinary muscular movement, such as is necessarily used in the daily avocations of life, or instinctively used in obedience to the imperative demand of the muscular sense, to maintain this normal movement of the cell contents.

"It is the function of 'remedial,' or 'localized,' or 'Swedish' movements and massage to restore this normal movement of the cell contents when it has become retarded or otherwise disarranged. This therapeutic method, therefore, addresses itself to the very beginnings of life and nutrition, building up the frame anew from the foundation; and hence it is that its reconstructive results are of so permanent a character. Founded upon the strictest inductions of science, and in harmony with the most recent revelations of physiological investigations, it stands upon a plane of certainty in theory, and of precision in practice, not attainable by the more empirical systems of the *materia medica*."

The system was arranged by Dr. Ling of Sweden, about ninety years ago. He studied the Greek gymnastics, together with those of the more modern nations, and tested the hygienic meaning of each movement. Those that tended to produce or encourage bad posture or other unfavorable influence upon health he discarded, also those of no distinct hygienic value, leaving but sixty elementary movements. He also tested each movement with respect to its influence on the heart action and lung power, and the strength of these two sets of organs formed the basis for the arrangement of his system.

The movements may be compared to the elementary sounds of our language, which, in their many combinations, make the thousands of words we use. So with the simple Swedish movements. Each movement gives little advantage by itself, but combined with those which precede and those which follow, brings the harmony of health for which we are aiming. For beginning exercises, simple movements in simple postures are arranged, progressing the work in a scientific and harmonious way as skill and physical vigor attained show need of more vigorous exercise. More difficult posture for the same movement is used, and more difficult movement for the same posture, until, in the progression that follows through months of work, complex movements in very difficult postures are given, bringing all the muscles and joints into coördination. Ling's followers claim that he was the originator of "systematized progressive gymnastics," not of the movements themselves.

This progression comprises the "Swedish system," which we employ in class exercise, and when no need presents itself other than symmetrical growth and development, and the promotion and preservation of health. The arrangement of the formula is also based on a scientific plan, and is never reversed, nor are movements omitted, so closely calculated is the influence produced by one class of movements upon that produced by another class.

The "system" is usually considered educational gymnastics. The Swedish work also covers the military; the recreative, or æsthetic; and the medical, or Swedish movements. The latter are employed when health is lacking and we desire to localize effects in the defective muscles. This localized work is the climax of the prescription, and is approached and followed by general work. It is usually passive, and accompanied by manipulations and massage.

Every Swedish movement is the embodiment of mechanical, psychological, and physiological laws, and should be clearly explained as such when recommended to the individual for practice. No one can thrive on mysteries; it is the right of every intelligent mind to understand his body, and know to what it is being subjected.

The mechanical laws embodied in the Swedish system are mainly those of leverage, resistance, and poise, or equilibrium. The physiological are those relating to organic, muscular, and nervous conditions. The psychological relate to the development of courage and skill, and to repose and will power, which are employed in localizing the energy to certain groups of muscles while isolating others; in fact, causing a muscle to follow the thought, or, as more commonly expressed, "willing a muscle."

Harmony, or health, as the word should be interpreted, is the outgrowth of these three applied sciences. In this book of preliminary body study they are but suggested. I will give a brief outline of the meaning of the different sets of movements, classified in their order.

RESPIRATORY MOVEMENT (often employed to introduce an order of practice): to raise the chest, open the lung cells and change the air contained in them, and to stimulate the spinal nerves.

FOOT MOVEMENT: to direct the blood current to the lower extremities, and to train for good poise and good carriage.

HEAD MOVEMENT: to localize energy in muscles of neck, and, by improving the circulation there, to render flexible the tissues, and prevent congestive conditions of head, eyes, ears, and throat; also to cultivate graceful poise of the head.

CHEST MOVEMENT: to raise the chest, and, consequently, the entire viscera; improve the muscles of the upper spine and the muscles of respiration, and to increase chest capacity.

SHOULDER-BLADE MOVEMENT: to localize work to the muscles of shoulders, upper spine, and chest; to improve the hand and arm muscles, and correct errors in position of shoulder-blades.

This and chest movements are considered by

many the true beginning movements; those that precede them being but preliminary.

BALANCE MOVEMENT: to cultivate good poise, skill, and muscular control, and to direct the blood current to the lower limbs, thereby relieving any blood pressure that may be experienced in the muscles recently employed.

BACK MOVEMENT: to strengthen system of spinal muscles, overcome the tendency to spinal deviation, if any exists, correct irregularities of posture, and stimulate the spinal nerves.

ABDOMINAL MOVEMENT: to strengthen the abdominal walls, correct the figure in case of sagging abdomen or superfluous adipose, and improve digestion.

LATERAL TRUNK MOVEMENT: to supplement the advantages specified in the abdominal movement, make flexible the intercostals, facilitate the current in inferior vena cava, improve portal and renal circulation, increase activity of liver and intestines, and stimulate spinal nerves. It develops "nature's corsets," as Baron Posse so aptly remarks.

These three sets of movements are the specific ones, and are only to be practiced when preceded and followed by work for the limbs.

JUMP MOVEMENT: to accelerate the blood current and cultivate skill and coördination. This is not to be employed for adults, except when their conditions are favorable for such active exercise.

LEG MOVEMENT: to use in place of the jump, or to follow it if the blood current has been accelerated unduly by the more energetic work and needs to be normalized.

RESPIRATORY MOVEMENT: to eliminate carbonic acid gas caused by the excess of exercise, to increase elasticity of chest walls and lung cells, to normalize the breathing, and bring repose. This should never be omitted.

This, in brief, is the translation of Ling's formula and definitions, by many Swedish leaders.

In adapting the work to the needs of American women and children, I adhere to his "system," but necessarily arrange posture and movement to suit American physique. Climatic influences, and the ravages mental pressure makes on nerve power, and particularly the inherent tendency to disease, make it impossible to use the Swedish system unconditionally for women. It is safe if begun in earlier years, as in schools, and continued throughout the growing period; but must be used with discretion in adult life, else unfavorable results are as liable to attend it as the less scientific plans of gymnastic work.

Many of the movements in these lessons for home practice are necessarily from recumbent posture, whether for adult or child. The adult needs a posture that normalizes the position of internal organs which from unhygienic influences have become depressed, a posture that makes tense the abdominal walls without causing downward pressure of the viscera, and one that relieves the spinal muscles from responsibility of good posture. The recumbent covers these requirements.

For the child, whose need is largely to have the chest raised and back muscles and abdominal walls strengthened, the recumbent posture offers the greatest advantage; because in standing, the errors of posture that have become second nature in daily life are liable to attend the practice of the movements, thus making them more harmful than advantageous.

For example: if a child habitually carries his head forward, chin raised, and the chest consequently lowered and abdomen protruded, it is evident that even the practice of a simple foot or arm movement would harden still more firmly the muscles in that abnormal position, while even these same simple exercises from good posture will help correct such faults. Parents and teachers should look carefully to posture of children in class gymnastics, and unless good attention is given to this essential, should discontinue all such exercises.

There should be as close observance given to accuracy in this as would be given in music practice; in fact, more, since we are aiming to produce harmony, and to dispel the physical discord that is filling our homes with semi-invalids.

The movements should be practiced slowly, never exciting the nerve centres, but using nerve strength evenly.

Practicing any gymnastic exercise to music is unwise, except in marching, dancing, club swinging, or other such rhythmic motion. In trunk movements, or other localized work, the value of the movement is lost in aiming to execute it within the limit of time allowed by the music. Through influence of the music we lose accuracy of movement and of posture, and we are also liable to omit the force necessary to be given in practice of extensor muscles, as in shoulder-blade movement.

Every group of muscles is antagonized by an opposing group. When these two groups are equally exercised, we say that their intermediate position is maintained. When one is habitually exercised in excess of the other, it becomes permanently shortened, and the opposing ones are permanently lengthened; the intermediate position is lost, and lack of harmony in figure or health, usually both, is the result. (The chapter on Spines clearly illustrates this fact.) It is necessary in such cases to ascertain where the disused muscles lie, and arrange localized gymnastic exercises to benefit them. We speak of localizing a movement when we direct the energy to certain groups of muscles. Isolation accompanies localization, and implies the ability to move out of certain groups of muscles or a member, as an arm or a foot. Coördination includes harmony of mind and muscle. These three are largely dependent upon psychological laws.

The hygienic and therapeutic value of a movement depends upon skill, and the energy and resistance employed in executing it. A convenient explanation of resistance is, forcing the strength against itself. Or, in other words, we hold the movement back with the muscles that oppose the ones employed in executing it, using sufficient resistance to steady the movement, and prevent its being rapid or jerky. Or, in further explanation, one set of muscles, the flexor, we will say, contracts to execute a movement, and the opposing set, the extensor, is employed to hinder the movement.

We speak of applied resistance when the individual applies resistive force, as pressing one hand against the other; or against the head, to resist a head movement; or when the opposing strength of another person is employed. Resistance is especially necessary in shoulder-blade movements. In some of the trunk movements, and those for the legs, the weight of the trunk offers the necessary resistance.

Natural resistance takes the place of light apparatus, such as pulley weights, Indian clubs, etc., and is preferable, if for no other than the following reasons, which must appeal to every thinking person, viz:

1. It trains will power and coördination.

2. It gives opportunity for the individual to discriminate in regard to expenditure of energy. Conditions and influences vary from day to day, and each one's outlay of energy should be adjusted to correspond with them.

3. It prevents cramping the hands, an argument of itself convincing, as every occupation of life tends to develop the flexor muscles of the hands, and in our gymnastic exercise we must direct our energies to the extensor muscles.

Bed-time is the period best calculated to bring good results in home gymnastics. The work rests the tired mind and muscles, and normalizes the circulation. Sleep is easily induced, and proves more restful than it would without the exercise. The period of rest which should follow, in order that the blood be not impeded in its circulation through tissues thus forced, comes at a favorable hour.

It is also of great advantage to practice in mid-day; luncheon is then an acceptable and salutary meal, especially if followed by a half hour of repose.

These exercises should never be practiced directly after eating. An hour after a light meal, or two hours after a heavier one, will be a sufficient interval. Repose should follow the practice so that good circulation will be allowed to continue in the unused tissues that are necessarily forced. Following customary habits too soon after the practice will, with delicate people, not only occasion fatigue, but much of the advantage gained by stimulating the disused muscles will thereby be lost.

From ten to forty minutes should be devoted to the work, and other interests should not be allowed to encroach upon this necessary care of the body. If, however, any emergency demands that the period of practice be shortened, let it be done by taking fewer repetitions of each movement, not by omitting any, or by hurrying through the entire schedule. Better omit it all than make it but a caricature. It is also unwise to select from the lessons the movements best calculated in the amateur's mind to improve conditions, and to neglect the practice of the others prescribed. This, I find, is the tendency in obesity, thin necks, or other undesirable conditions where beauty rather than health is involved. The work is necessarily localized in these defective muscles, but general work is imperative with the specific, not alone for harmony of health, but to draw excess of blood away from the weak tissues, after having forced it through them by the localized exercise. Our aim is health, and unless rational means are employed in securing it, the attempt will not prove successful.

Soreness may follow the early practice, but it need occasion no anxiety. In the resistance of unused muscles it is often a result. As the muscles become trained to contractility and flexibility it will disappear; hence accept it as an accompaniment of muscle growth, and continue the practice.

These formulæ are arranged for average conditions of heart action and pelvic health. Discretion should be used in regard to both posture and movement, although the beginning lessons are very simple. Individual resources, conditions, and age must also enter into the arrangement of work, and limitations of strength must never be reached.

Loose, comfortable clothing should always be worn during practice. A gymnasium suit is of itself an inspiration.

If the work is being directed for others, as by the mother for her children, the orders should be given in slow intonations, yet using force. A military command encourages spasmodic movement, and this we desire to avoid. American nerves need a sedative, not an accelerator, and hence influences of an exciting nature should be avoided. "Breathe freely, practice slowly and resistively," should be every one's motto. In the gymnasium, speed is often recommended; but in this first volume of home exercise we will give it no explanation, except the jump movement, and instead, I will emphasize the request to practice slowly. In this way every one is benefited, and nervous or delicate people are not injured, as they probably would be by rapid movements. Each position should be held from three to five heart-beats, breathing freely, but not heavily, meanwhile, in order to allow the blood current to do its work while muscles are placed on a stretch.

A few minutes' repose should be allowed between the different sets of exercises.

The numbers at the right of described movements indicate the number of repetitions for each. 5–8 means that five repetitions are for beginning practice, and that they are to be increased in number, at discretion, until eight are reached.

The descriptions are given in the fewest possible words, and are literal. I have had the movements interpreted by several women unversed in the science, and each time a clear comprehension of the text was shown; hence I feel satisfied that the lessons are clearly rendered.

An illustration of each posture will accompany the description, and reference will be made to the same by number when it is introduced into subsequent lessons.

It is advantageous to practice before a mirror; it will aid in accuracy.

Use the muscles on the left side before using those on the right; it aids in cultivating ambidexterity.

Every movement will include the thought, the action, and the return to the medium position, which we consider normalizing the muscles that have been employed.

This work has been arranged for the average American woman and girl. The plan is the outgrowth of many years of experience throughout both North and South, and with all types of physique. My work has always been characterized by a careful individual study of conditions, and has at no time been experimental. In this book I cannot, of course, give individual directions, but enough of theory is placed here to enable the careful reader to adapt the prescriptions to her needs. (For further advice see chapter on Diagnosis.)

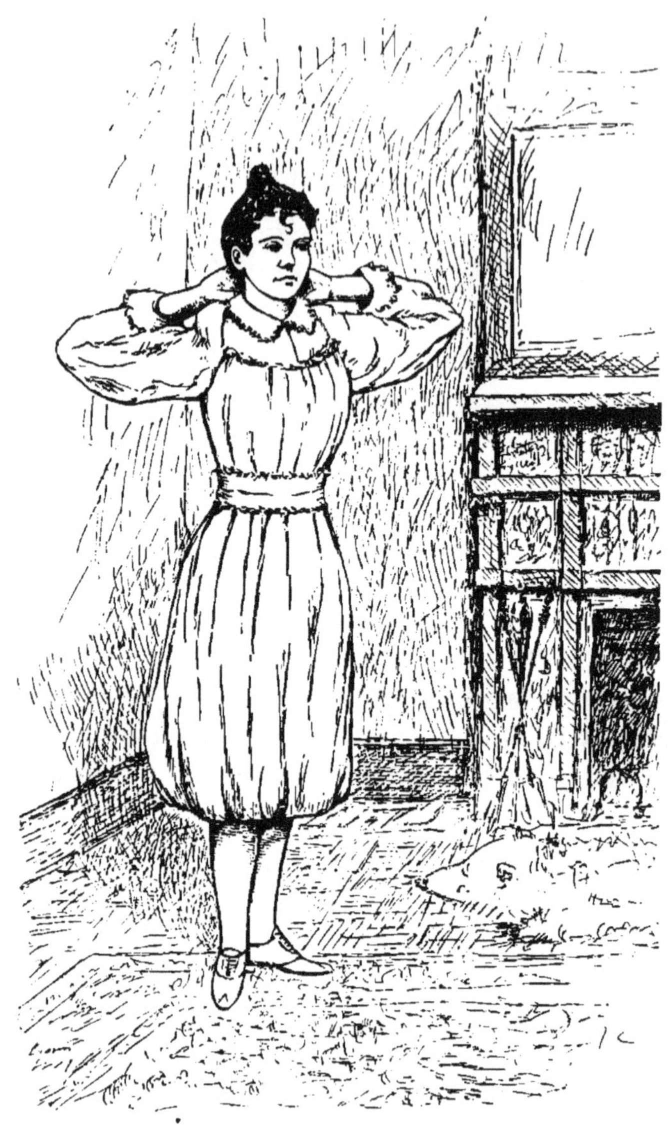

XXIII.

CHAPTER IX

SWEDISH EXERCISE FOR HOME PRACTICE

"Nobody is healthy without exercise."—ALEYN.

LESSON I.—ADULTS. FOR ONE WEEK'S PRACTICE

POSTURE must be our first study.

Correct posture brings the chest and abdomen in direct line, and the centre of weight of the trunk over the bones of the legs. This is attained by raising the chest and drawing back the hips, not by drawing back the shoulders and drawing in the abdomen. In this way the pubic arch is carried back of the line of the clavicular notch, and natural equilibrium is attained (see chapter on Spine). We train the muscles, in standing, always from this posture, with head erect, chin drawn slightly in, weight resting alike on each foot, feet at an angle of ninety degrees, weight of arms brought to bear on shoulder-blades, not on chest. We maintain this posture during intervals of practice, but it is essential that rigidity of muscle be avoided. The energy must be directed to the groups of muscles employed, isolating others, or rather using others automatically only, in maintaining good posture. It is not easy to *move out* of unemployed members, as in our American haste we have become accustomed to keeping all our powers on the alert; but this ability once attained, will prove a powerful agent in the economy of health.

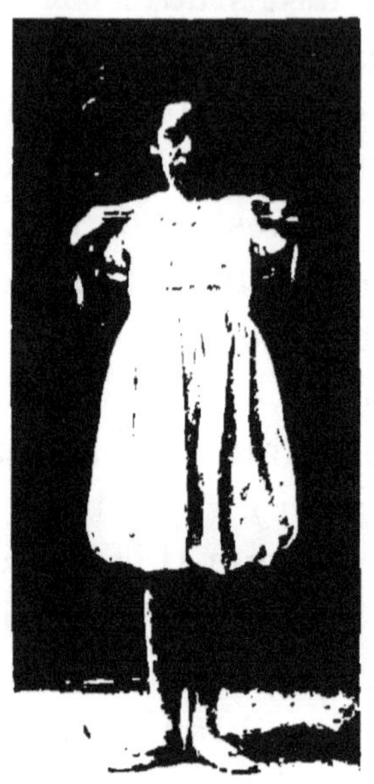

XXIV.

RESPIRATORY MOVEMENT.—Bend posture; *i. e.*, arms upward bend, finger tips touching shoulders; the movement involves raising the elbows shoulder high and at the same time inhaling; then lowering them to former position, exhaling. (10 repetitions.) Care must be taken that elbows are not brought to the front in this movement; weight of arms must be suspended from back of the body. Make inhalations through the nose, exhalations through the mouth, in all respiratory movements. Should this deep breathing cause dizziness, the following foot movement will doubtless allay it.

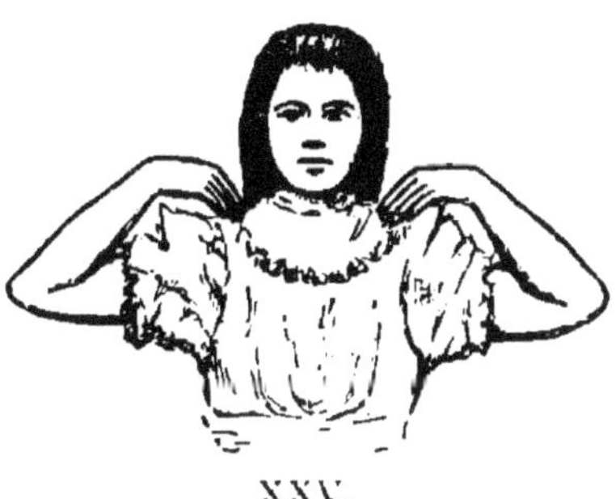

XXV.

Foot Movement. —Hips firm; *i. e.*, hands on hips, thumbs backward, hand and arm in line; *heels raise; i. e.*, a slow raise on toes, feet to maintain angle of ninety degrees; hold posture until good balance is attained; *heels sink; i. e.*, to slowly assume first position. (10 repetitions.)

Remember to execute it slowly; a jerky movement not only makes good muscular control impossible, but destroys repose, which means also destruction of grace and endurance.

This foot movement is repeated frequently to draw the blood to the lower members.

Head Movement. — Standing or sitting erect; *head to left twist*, slowly and with slight resistance; *head forward twist.* (3–5 or 8 repetitions.) The same movement to the right. Do not tip the head in executing the movement. Hold opposing neck muscles firm, not rigid, in resisting the movement. Tense neck muscles destroy beauty by causing deep lines.

SHOULDER-BLADE MOVEMENT.—*Arm rotation.* (8–12 repetitions.) Make tense all extensor muscles of the arm and hand; turn arms from position of palms against the body outward, making the strongest pull with muscles of shoulder-blades. Relax muscles slowly, and allow arms to resume first position. This movement practiced from position of arms raised to shoulder height (posture XXXIV.) will occasion more energy to be directed to shoulder-blade muscles, hence is an advance in progression.

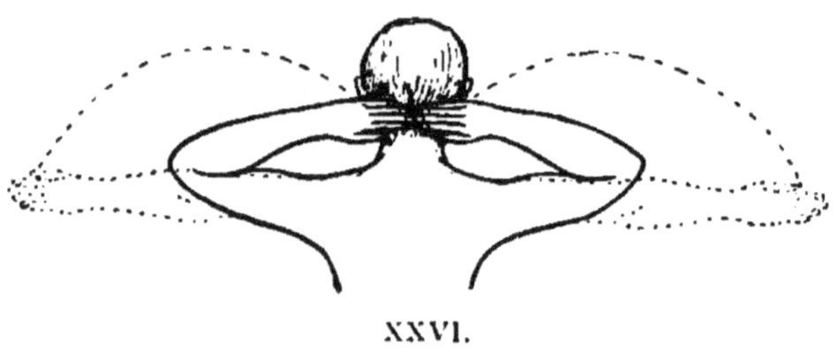

XXVI.

FOOT MOVEMENT. — Repeat the one described above, from *neck firm* position. To gain this position, raise arms to plane of shoulders, flex elbows, and bring finger-tips in touch, not clasped, at back of neck (posture XXVI.).

The circulation, by these exercises, will have been well stimulated in the extremities, hence the system is in readiness for the trunk movements.

BACK MOVEMENT.—Standing or stride-sitting, *i. e.*, knees at an angle of ninety degrees; hips firm; *trunk forward bend.* (5–10 repetitions.) The movement is from the hips only, and the muscles of the spine must be held tense in carrying the trunk forward; take care to hold the face in its former plane, so that the muscles of the upper spine are correctly employed, and chest posture is improved.

ABDOMINAL MOVEMENT.—Recumbent posture; neck firm; *leg raise.* (3-8 repetitions.) Begin this movement by extending the foot in line with the leg, and at first only willing the muscles to be employed in raising the leg. Execute the movement at discretion, keeping the knee muscles tense, raising the foot but a few inches, and resuming former posture slowly, never suddenly. Relax the muscles for momentary rest, and repeat the movement.

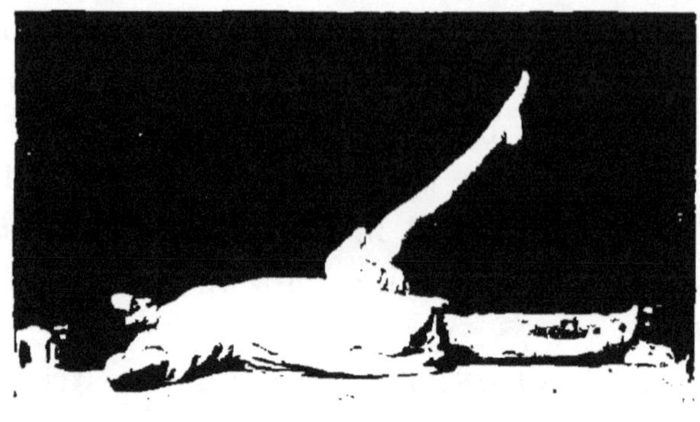

XXVII.

Much harm may result to the abdominal organs by practicing this movement indiscriminately. Forty-five degrees is a sufficient angle,

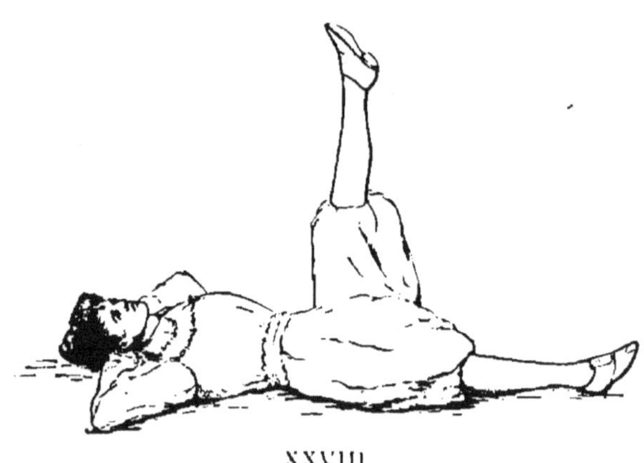

XXVIII

even for flexible muscles; but in cases of good muscular control, ninety degrees may be reached. In no wise attempt legs raise simultaneously until weeks of practice on this milder movement warrant it a safe procedure. In case of pelvic weakness, this class of movements should not be practiced, except on advice from the physician.

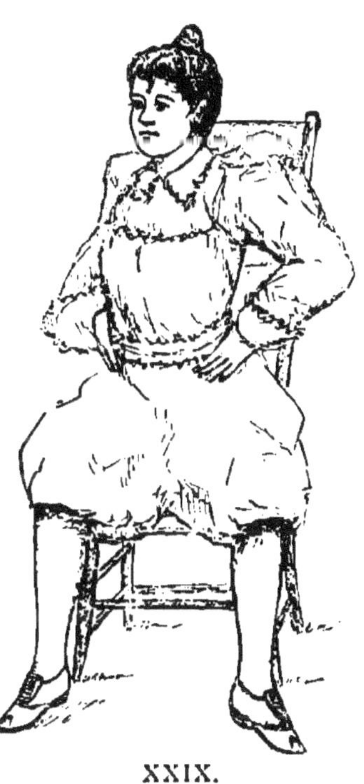

XXIX.

SIDE MOVEMENT.—Stride-sitting; hips firm; *trunk to left twist.* (5–8 repetitions.) Same to right side. The energy is directed to the intercostals, and the movement is performed in the main by them, although the transverse muscles of the abdomen, and the spinal muscles give secondary aid. The trunk moves on the pelvis; hip joints are not employed. This movement should not be practiced from standing posture until the muscles named obey the will. Good chest posture must be maintained. Breathe freely, but not in rhythm with the movement.

FOOT MOVEMENT.—Repeat the first foot movement.

RESPIRATORY MOVEMENT.—Repeat the first respiratory movement.

MEMORANDUM OF LESSON I

Adults

Respiratory Movement.—Arms bend; *elbows raise, inhaling.* (10 repetitions.)

Foot Movement.—Hips firm; *heels raise.* (10 repetitions.)

Head Movement.—Sitting; *head twist.* (3–5 repetitions.)

Shoulder-blade Movement.—*Arm rotation.* (12 repetitions.)

Balance Movement.—Neck firm; *heels raise.* (10 repetitions.)

Back Movement.—Stride-sitting or standing; hips firm; *trunk forward bend.* (5–8 repetitions.)

Abdominal Movement.—Recumbent posture; hips firm or neck firm; *leg raise.* (3–8 repetitions.)

Side Movement.—Stride-sitting; hips firm; *trunk twist.* (5–8 repetitions.)

Foot Movement.—Hips firm or neck firm; *heels raise.* (10 repetitions.)

Respiratory Movement.—As first.

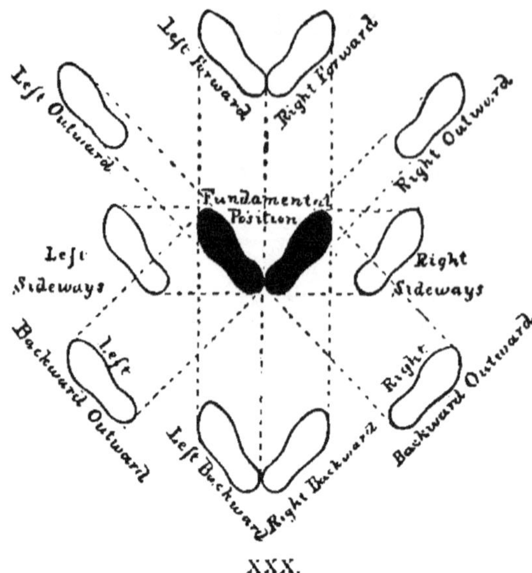

XXX.

FOOT CHART.

This shows the direction of angle in different foot-placing gymnastics; the training in these is a strong power in cultivating repose in posture and ease of carriage, if the chest is raised, and thought is used to keep the weight balanced equally on both feet.

CHAPTER X

SWEDISH EXERCISE FOR HOME PRACTICE

(Continued)

"Physic, for the most part, is nothing else but the substitute for exercise and temperance."—ADDISON.

LESSON II.—ADULTS

EACH lesson is for one week or more of practice, and should be continued until muscular ability is attained, and more vigorous exercise can be discreetly undertaken.

When no mention of posture is made, fundamental standing position is meant.

RESPIRATORY MOVEMENT.—*Arms sideways raise, inhaling; downward sink, exhaling.* (10 repetitions.) Arms should be in direct line of shoulder-blades.

FOOT MOVEMENT.—Hips firm; *foot forward place* (3 repetitions for each foot); also *foot backward place.* (3 repetitions.)

The step is twice the length of the foot; the trunk is carried forward with it and rests proportionately on both feet; the chest is carried forward in its own plane. (See foot chart.) Avoid twisting or inclining the trunk, or protruding the abdomen. This foot-placing movement is invaluable as an aid in graceful carriage and repose in walking. If either foot can be raised without changing the weight to the other, it is evident that the body is not equally poised on both, hence the posture is incorrect.

HEAD MOVEMENT.—Standing or sitting; hips firm; *head sideways bend*, slowly and with slight resistance; *upward raise*. (3 8 repetitions.)

Take care that chin is not raised, and that opposing muscles are not rigid.

SHOULDER-BLADE MOVEMENT.—Standing or sitting; arms sideways raise; and from that position, *arm circling*. (5–12 repetitions.)

Keep extensor muscles well stretched, and make the circle entirely at side and back of trunk, employing primarily the muscles that control the shoulder-blades. Or, to be more clear, make the circle up, back, and down, not toward the front. The same movement is made more vigorous by practicing from palms up (posture LIV., chapter XIII.).

BALANCE MOVEMENT. — Neck firm; left foot forward place, carrying the trunk forward, and supporting its weight equally on both feet (notice directions given in foot movement); from this step posture, *heels raise;* pause until perfect balance is attained; *heels sink* (5 repetitions); foot replace, carrying weight of the trunk with the foot. Same movement, advancing the right foot. (5 repetitions.)

Practice also from foot backward place.

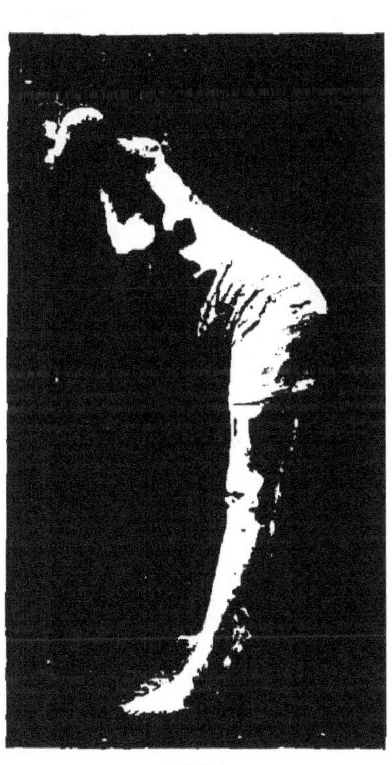

XXXI.

BACK MOVEMENT.—Stride-standing or stride-sitting; neck firm; *trunk forward bend.* (5 10 repetitions.)

Give careful attention to holding the chest high and the face in its former plane during the movement, so that muscles of the upper spine are well employed.

ABDOMINAL MOVEMENT.—Recumbent posture; neck firm; *leg raise;* hold posture during a few heart-beats: *leg sink.* (5-8 repetitions.) Outlined in lesson I.; use discretion in repetitions and height of angle.

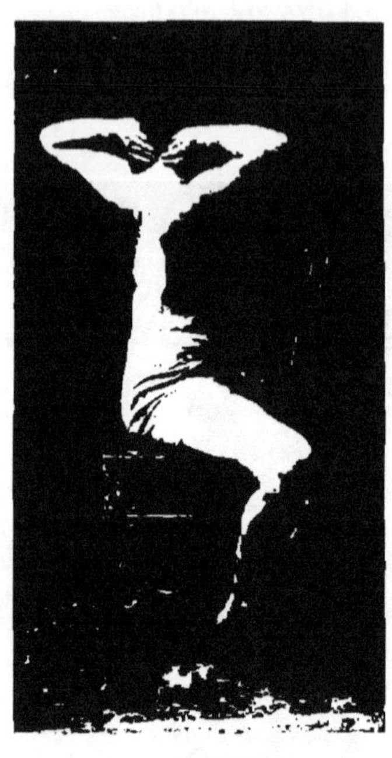

XXXII.

Muscular control is proved by steadiness of slow movement. Be careful to keep the foot in extension.

SIDE MOVEMENT.—Sitting; neck firm; *trunk twist.* (5–8 repetitions.) Described in first week's practice; the movement is made more vigorous by posture XXXII. The head should follow the plane of the chest, not turn in advance of it. The effort is localized in the intercostals. This is invaluable in improving condition of digestive apparatus. (See definition of side movement in chapter on Swedish Exercise for Home Practice.)

FOOT MOVEMENT.—Neck firm; *heels raise.* (10 repetitions.)

RESPIRATORY MOVEMENT.—As at beginning of this lesson.

Or, from recumbent, half-lying, or hook-lying posture (see lesson of Recumbent Posture Movements), arms upward bend; *arm extension in line with trunk, at same time inhaling, resume bend position of arms while exhaling.* (10 repetitions.)

Remain in recumbent position for rest.

MEMORANDUM OF LESSON II

Adults

Respiratory Movement.—*Arms sideways raise, inhaling; downward sink, exhaling.* (10 repetitions.)

Foot Movement.—Hips firm; *foot forward place;* also *backward place.* (3 repetitions each.)

Head Movement.—Standing or sitting; hips firm; *head to side bend.* (5–8 repetitions.)

Shoulder-blade Movement.—Arms sideways raise; *arm cirling.* (5–12 repetitions.)

Or, same, from palms held upward.

Balance Movement.—Neck firm; foot forward place; *heels raise.* (5 repetitions.)

Back Movement.—Stride-standing or stride-sitting; neck firm; *trunk forward bend.* (5–8 repetitions.)

Abdominal Movement.—Lying; neck firm; *leg raise.* (3–8 repetitions.)

Side Movement.—Stride-sitting (facing chair-back); neck firm; *trunk twist.* (8 repetitions.)

Leg Movement.—Neck firm; *heels raise.* (10 repetitions.)

Respiratory Movement.—As beginning movement. (10 repetitions.)

Or, lying; *arm extension in line with trunk.* (10 repetitions.)

CHAPTER XI

SWEDISH EXERCISE FOR HOME PRACTICE
(*Continued*)

"Activity does not mean excitement. Healthful action is uniform."—BRINTON.

LESSON III.—ADULTS

RESPIRATORY MOVEMENT.—As lesson II. (10 repetitions.)

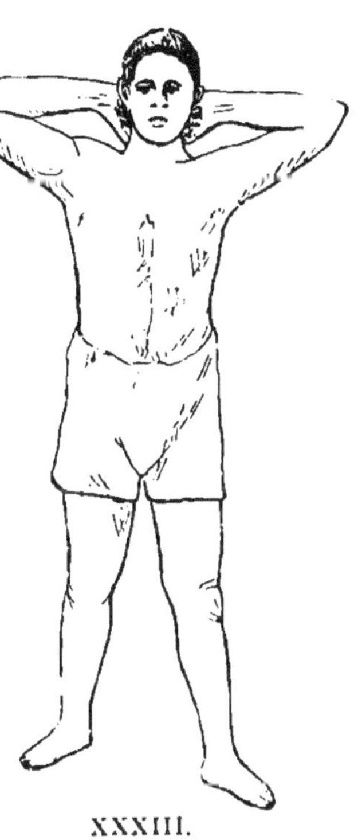

XXXIII.

FOOT MOVEMENT.—Neck firm: *foot outward place.* (5 repetitions each.)

Carry the foot in its own direction, about twice its length. (See foot chart XXX.)

Care must be exercised to carry the trunk in the direction of the foot placing; maintain good chest posture; avoid protruding the abdomen or twisting the trunk, and be careful to support the weight equally on both feet.

Practice also backward-outward placing of foot; *i. e.*, directing the movement diagonally backward in line of the other foot. Observe carefully the cautions mentioned. These movements are invaluable if accurately practiced.

HEAD MOVEMENT.—From lesson I. or II.; *i. e., head twist* or *bend.* (8 repetitions.)

SHOULDER-BLADE MOVEMENT.—Arms upward bend (see posture XXIV., lesson I.), resisting shoulder-blade muscles; turn hands around, toward the front, to the side; *arms sideways stretch;* make the movement resistive until the limit of arm extension is complete, and then aim to reach a point beyond the possible stretch. This enforced mus-

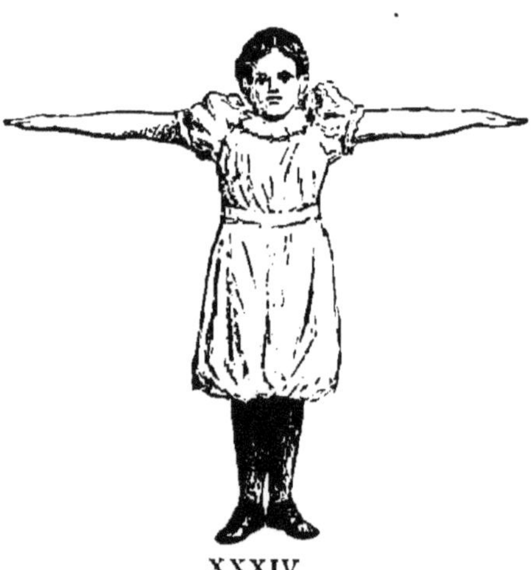

XXXIV.

cle extension gives the movement especial value. The return to former position is also a resistive movement, and is as follows: *arms bend* resistively; hands turn downward; *arms downward stretch* resistively to first position. (5–8 repetitions of the entire movement.)

These practiced properly bring circulation through extensor muscles of arms and hands, and are invaluable for chest and shoulder muscles. Good breathing, and accuracy in posture and execution must be observed.

FOOT MOVEMENT.—Recumbent posture; neck firm; *bend and stretch ankles.* (10–20 repetitions.) This movement must be slow and resistive, maintaining the ninety degrees angle of feet. The effort is localized in the extremities. It is a restful movement, and is introduced frequently for the purpose of directing the blood current to the lower limbs, and thus relieving pressure in the head.

BACK MOVEMENT.—Chest-lying; hips firm; feet fixed; *i. e.*, placed under a piece of heavy furniture for support, or held firmly by an attendant (postures XXXV. and XXXVI.); *head and shoulders raise.* (5–8 repetitions.)

The movement must begin with raising the

head; the shoulder muscles are next involved, and then the muscles of the lower spine. Use care that elbows do not droop.

The posture is more difficult than any in the preceding lessons, consequently be careful not to hold the breath. In returning to rest posi-

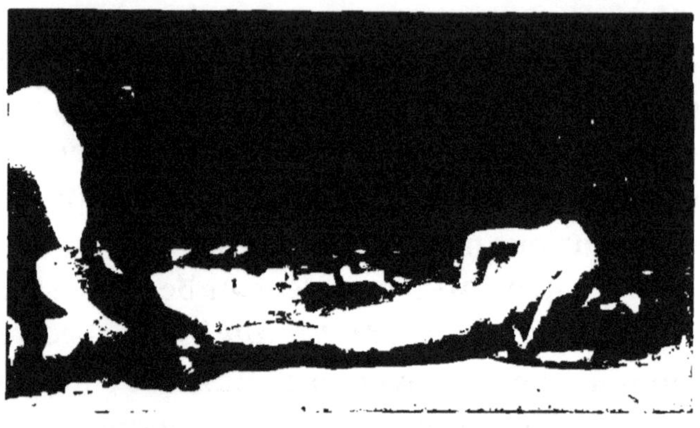

XXXV.

tion, relax first the lower spinal muscles, then those controlling the shoulders, and finally those of the neck. The movement is a difficult one, and should be very discreetly practiced. With the majority of women, unused to gymnastic exercise, merely the head and shoulders should be raised in the beginning weeks of practice, and progression must be discreetly conducted. Posture XXXVI. may not be safe in months of practice.

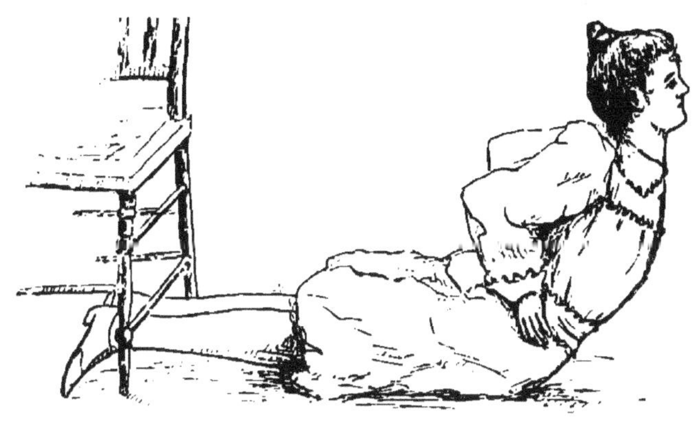

XXXVI.

Abdominal Movement.—Recumbent posture; hips firm; extend ankles and raise leg (see posture XXVII., lesson I.); *leg circumduction; i. e.* wide circle from hip. (3–8 repetitions.)

Make the circumduction outward, and direct the thought to the extremities, using great force in the extensor muscles.

Side Movement. — Standing or sitting; neck firm; *trunk sideways bend.* (5–8 repetitions.)

This movement should be made directly to the side; tipping to the back might cause strain on abdominal walls, and would certainly prove harmful to good posture, as would also tipping to the front. Mobility in joints of lower limbs should be avoided. The movement is made largely with the intercostals, those on the flexed side shortening as much as possible, and those on the opposite side stretching correspondingly. The bellows of the accordeon make a clear illustration of this.

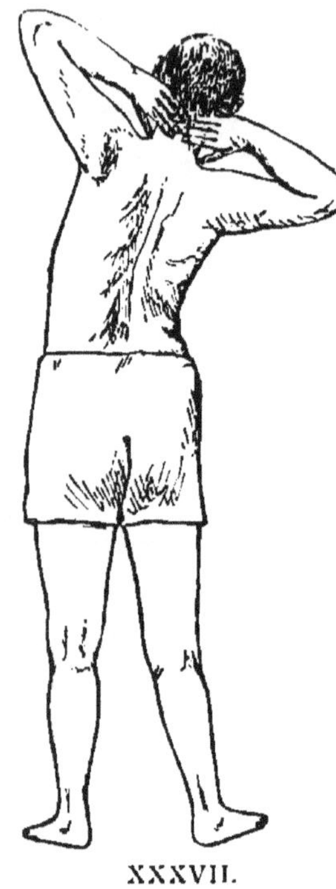

XXXVII.

Great advantage comes to lung tissue through improving the flexibility of chest walls.

Leg Movement.—Neck firm; stride-standing; *heels raise.* (10 repetitions.)

Or, recumbent posture; neck firm; *foot circumduction.* (12–15 repetitions.) First flex ankles, and then direct circumduction outward, making heavy stretch in the foot extension. The movement should be slow and resistive.

RESPIRATORY MOVEMENT.—*Arms sideways raise, inhaling; downward sink, exhaling.* (10 repetitions.)

Or, *arm extension*, from recumbent posture; the movements described in lesson II.

MEMORANDUM OF LESSON III

ADULTS

RESPIRATORY MOVEMENT.—*Arms sideways raise, inhaling.* (10 repetitions.)

FOOT MOVEMENT.—Neck firm; *foot outward place;* also *backward-outward place.* (3 repetitions each.)

HEAD MOVEMENT.—*Head bend,* or *head twist.* (8 repetitions.)

SHOULDER-BLADE MOVEMENT.—*Arms upward bend and sideways stretch; bend and downward stretch.* (5 repetitions.)

FOOT MOVEMENT.—Lying; neck firm; *bend and stretch ankles.* (10 repetitions.)

BACK MOVEMENT.—Chest-lying; feet fixed; *head and shoulders raise.* (5–8 repetitions.)

ABDOMINAL MOVEMENT.—Lying; neck firm; *leg circumduction.* (3–8 repetitions.)

SIDE MOVEMENT.—Standing or sitting; neck firm; *trunk to side, bend.* (5–8 repetitions.)

LEG MOVEMENT.—Neck firm; *heels raise.* (10 repetitions.)

Or, lying; neck firm; *feet circumduction.* (10 repetitions.)

RESPIRATORY MOVEMENT.—*Arms sideways raise, inhaling.* (10 repetitions.)

Or, lying; *arm extension in line with trunk.* (10 repetitions.)

CHAPTER XII

PRESCRIPTIONS OF EXERCISE FOR HOME PRACTICE

"O blessed health! thou art above all golden treasure."—STERNE.

PRESCRIPTION I.—ADULTS

THE practice of the foregoing lessons of elementary movements and simple postures will have prepared the way for the adapting of these to conditions, and also for more vigorous work.

The following lessons will take somewhat the form of prescriptions of exercise, and for convenience sake I will call them such.

In case of especially weak tissues, massage should be used in connection with the movements. The memoranda will refer to manipulations described in the chapter on Massage. These give more speedy relief than the movements do, but do not afford the desired advantage for tissue building and consequent permanent benefit.

In case of weak pelvic organs, the movements should be practiced from recumbent postures; but it is always best to have able advice before practicing any movements that would affect these organs, providing weak conditions are present.

RESPIRATORY MOVEMENT.—*Arms sideways raise, inhaling; downward sink, exhaling.* (10 repetitions.)

FOOT MOVEMENT.—Neck firm; *foot forward place; heels raise;* hold balance until full control of muscles is attained; *heels sink; foot replace.* (5 repetitions each.)

On alternate days practice same from foot backward place. There will be a tendency to incline the trunk backward in this, hence use care to maintain fundamental position of chest and trunk.

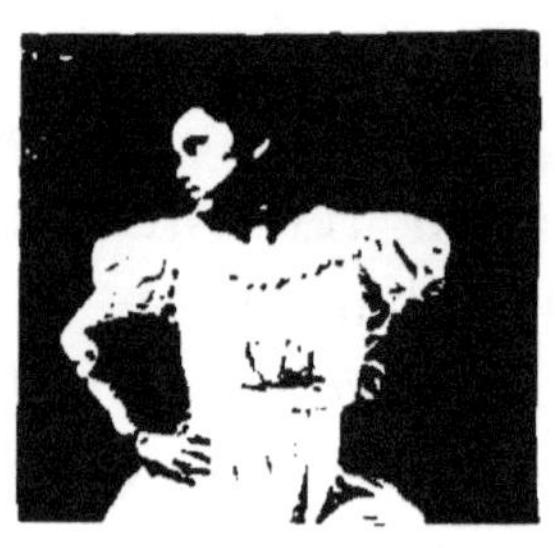

XXXVIII.

HEAD MOVEMENT.—Standing or sitting; hips firm; head twist; from this position, *head bend* to same side (posture XXXVIII.). (8 repetitions each side.)

Do not relax muscles used for twist posture

while taking bend movements; guard against rigidity of opposing muscles. Massage for weak or overtaxed organs of the head and throat, catarrhal affections, and colds, should follow head movements.

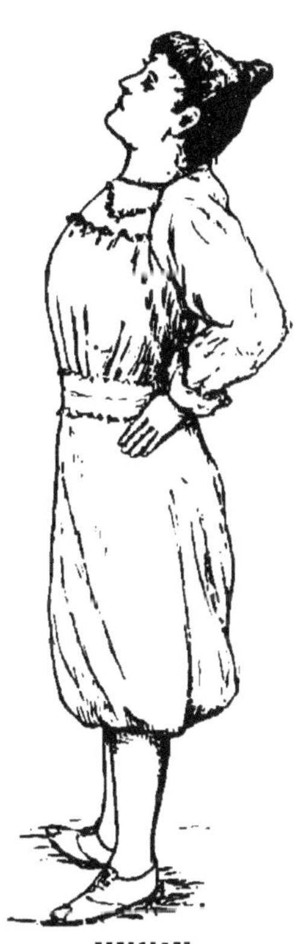

XXXIX.

CHEST MOVEMENT.—Standing or stride-sitting; hips firm; *head and upper spine backward bend.* (5–8 repetitions.) Keep the chin well drawn in, to avoid lax condition of front of neck, holding muscles firm, but not rigid.

Take care not to bend backward sharply at the waist. Always begin the arch by carrying the head backward, bringing leverage gradually on upper vertebræ, approaching lower at discretion. At no time allow hips (consequently abdomen) to protrude. This is properly named "chest raising," and if accurately executed, not only the chest, but the abdomen is raised, relieving the pelvis from downward pressure of abdominal viscera, and excellent results are sure to follow

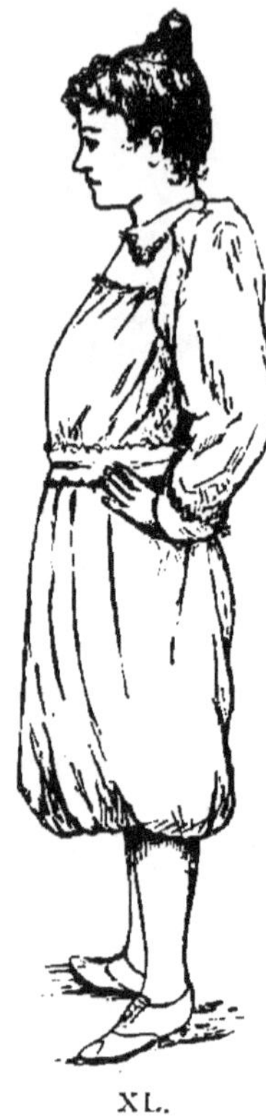

XL.

from normalizing the position of internal organs. On the other hand, much harm results from its being incorrectly practiced; if the chest is not raised according to directions, no advantage can come, and much harm to internal organs may follow. If the angle is directly from the waist backward, too great leverage is brought to bear on vertebræ at waist, and too heavy stretch is placed on the abdominal walls. Harm to spine, muscles, and organs results.

I wish, in behalf of the children in class practice, to call attention of mothers and teachers to this fact. I have seen the work executed many times as is represented in posture XL. Much more advantage results from practicing this movement from neck firm posture, as recommended in prescription III., but it should be approached at discretion.

In case of headache at base of brain, substitute for this movement the following: chest-lying; *upward raise;* the back movement described in lesson III. (5-8 repetitions.) Rotation or percussion of chest follows chest-raising when it is required.

SHOULDER-BLADE MOVEMENT.—*Arms sideways, upward, and downward stretch; i. e.*, arms

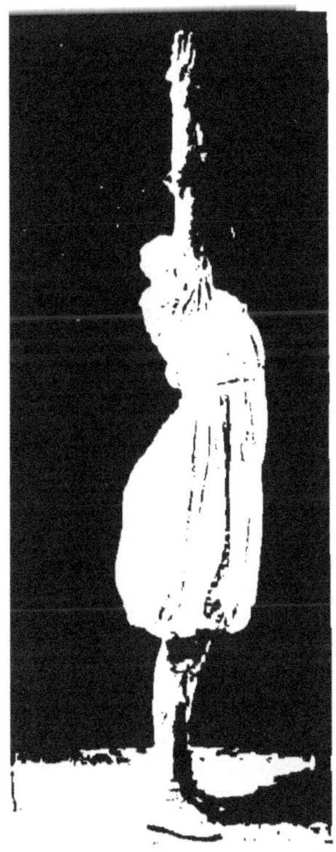

XLI.

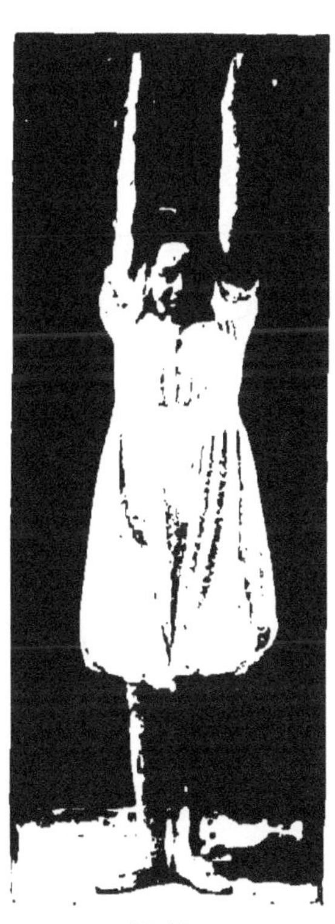

XLII.

bend and sideways stretch. (3–8 repetitions.) Described in lesson III. Resume bend position of arms; direct hands upward, and make a resistive upward stretch, raising elbows in side plane, not toward the front, and forcing

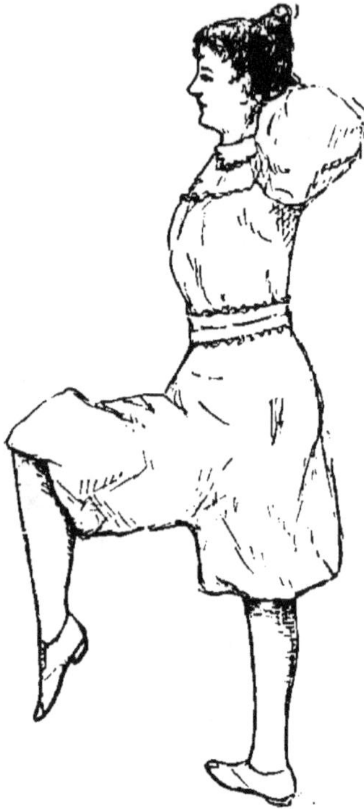

XLIII.—Balance Movement.

the stretch. After limit is reached, resume bend position, and execute the downward stretch as described in lesson III. Keep the palms directed toward each other, hands shoulder width apart, and take care that the head does not push forward in the upward stretch; this is a very valuable movement. In the chest elevation, and complete stretch of spinal muscles, the entire viscera is raised, and the system is strengthened for the more vigorous apparatus work, as suspending by arms from the horizontal bar, etc., often used for children.

Balance Movement.—Neck firm; *knee upward bend* (thigh and leg at right angles, foot extended, posture XLIII.); *forward stretch;* approach right angle at discretion (see posture LVIII., prescription III.); *forward-downward place,* walking slowly forward, carrying weight of trunk evenly. (10 to 20 steps.) Practice this with a book or other easily movable object on the head, to insure steady movement.

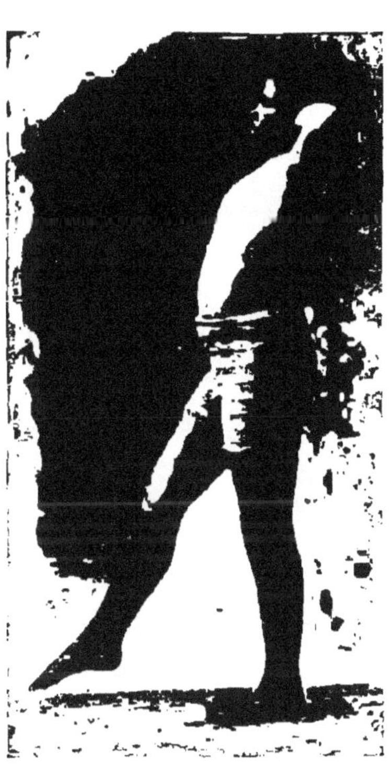

XLIV.

Pause between changes in posture for good poise.

Back Movement.—Chest-lying; feet fixed; hips firm; head and upper spine upward raise (posture XXXV., lesson III.); *head twist* alternately. (3–8 repetitions.)

Remember to keep the movement slow and steady. For alternate days, the same trunk posture; arms upward bend; *arms sideways stretch.* (3 repetitions.) Assume rest posture

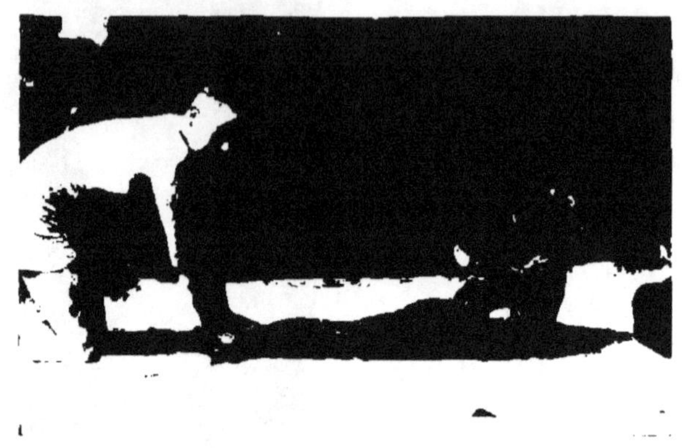

XLV.

for a few moments, and then raise the trunk and repeat the movement. (3 repetitions.) Increase repetitions at discretion to 5, possibly 8. Care should be taken that the head does not droop, that the muscles of shoulders and upper spine are held firm, and that chest is well arched. This movement should be practiced slowly.

In case muscles of upper spine are most in need of improvement, the head rotation affords the better advantage; if shoulder-blades, more advantage is gained through the arm stretch. Massage to be employed according to needs.

ABDOMINAL MOVEMENT.—Lying; neck firm; *leg circumduction.* (5–8 repetitions.) (See lesson III.)

Manipulation for stomach or liver.

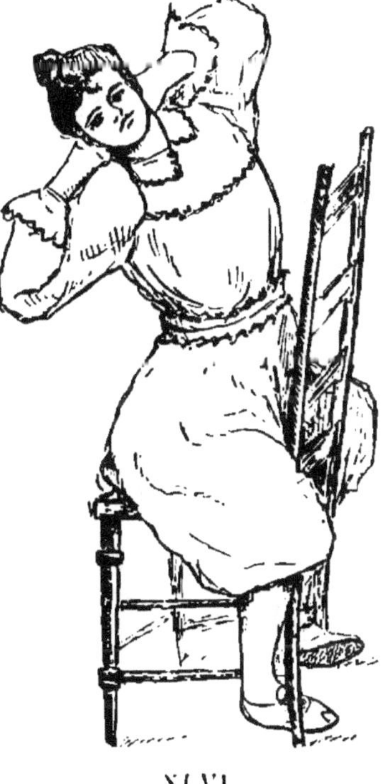

XLVI.

LATERAL TRUNK MOVEMENT.— Stride-sitting (feet locked around chair-legs); hips firm or neck firm at discretion; trunk twist; from this posture *trunk bend* to the same side. (5–8 repetitions to the left side, and the same to the right.)

Hold twist posture during repetitions of bend movement, taking care not to allow the chest to droop. Too great care regarding accuracy cannot be shown. The twist must not involve hip joints, and the bend must be directly under the arm-pit, not to the front nor to the back. Maintain good breathing, but do not have the breathing in unison with trunk movement.

Manipulate colon in case of constipation caused by lack of power in the digestive apparatus, and also increase number of repetitions of the movement. (See chapter on Diagnosis.)

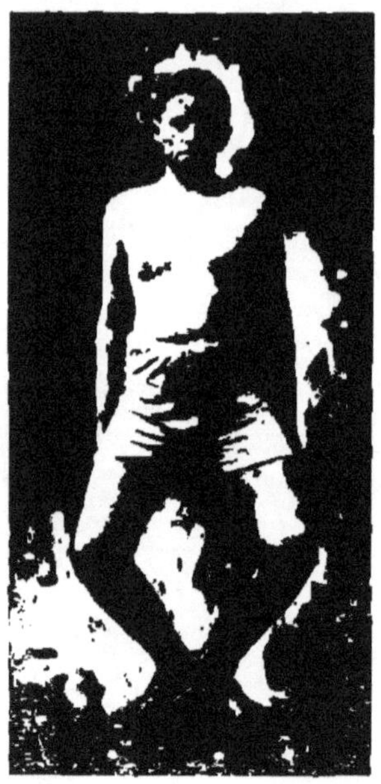

XLVII.

LEG MOVEMENT. — Hips firm; *heels raise; knees bend;* hold balance until complete muscular control is attained; *knees stretch; heels sink.* (3–10 repetitions.) In this toe-knee-bend-stand position, keep the heels in touch, knees at same angle as feet; *i.e.*, ninety degrees, and maintain fundamental position of the trunk.

This movement should be omitted in cases of pelvic weakness.

RESPIRATORY MOVEMENT.—Arms upward bend; *arm extension upward, inhaling; arms bend, exhaling.* (10 repetitions.)

Take care to maintain fundamental position of head and chest in this movement.

The arm extension brings the arms in the position of cuts XLI. and XLII., hands shoulder width apart, and palms toward each other. Correctly practiced, it is a valuable movement, but the advantage is lost if good posture is not maintained.

MEMORANDUM OF PRESCRIPTION I

Adults

RESPIRATORY MOVEMENT.—*Arms sideways raise, inhaling.* (10 repetitions.)

FOOT MOVEMENT.—Neck firm; foot forward place; *heels raise.* (3 repetitions each foot.) Also from foot backward place.

HEAD MOVEMENT.—Head twist; and to the same side *bend.* (3–8 repetitions.)

CHEST MOVEMENT.—Hips firm; *head and upper spine backward bend.* (5–8 repetitions.)

SHOULDER-BLADE MOVEMENT.—*Arms upward bend and sideways stretch; bend and upward stretch; bend and downward stretch.* (3–5 repetitions.)

FOOT MOVEMENT.—Neck firm; *knee upward bend; forward stretch; forward-downward place* (walking). (10–20 steps.)

BACK MOVEMENT.—Chest-lying; feet fixed; head and shoulders raise; *head rotation.* (3–8 repetitions.)

Or, from same posture, *arm extension sideways* (3 repetitions); rest, and repeat movement.

ABDOMINAL MOVEMENT.—Lying; neck firm; *leg circumduction.* (5–8 repetitions.)

LATERAL TRUNK MOVEMENT.—Stride-sitting; feet fixed; hips firm or neck firm; trunk twist; from that position *bend.* (3–8 repetitions.)

LEG MOVEMENT.—Hips firm; *heels raise; knees bend;* hold; *knees stretch; heels sink.* (3–8 repetitions.)

RESPIRATORY MOVEMENT.—Arms bend; *arm extension upward with deep breathing.* (10 repetitions.)

Massage should accompany the movements as directed in the prescription.

CHAPTER XIII

PRESCRIPTIONS OF EXERCISE FOR HOME PRACTICE (*Continued*)

"The wise for cure on exercise depend."

PRESCRIPTION II.—ADULTS. MORE VIGOROUS THAN THE FOREGOING

RESPIRATORY MOVEMENT.—*Arms sideways raise, inhaling; downward sink, exhaling.* (10 repetitions.)

FOOT MOVEMENT.—Neck firm; *foot outward place* (posture XXXIII., lesson III.); *heels raise;* hold poise until good muscular control is attained; *heels sink; foot replace.* (5 repetitions.)

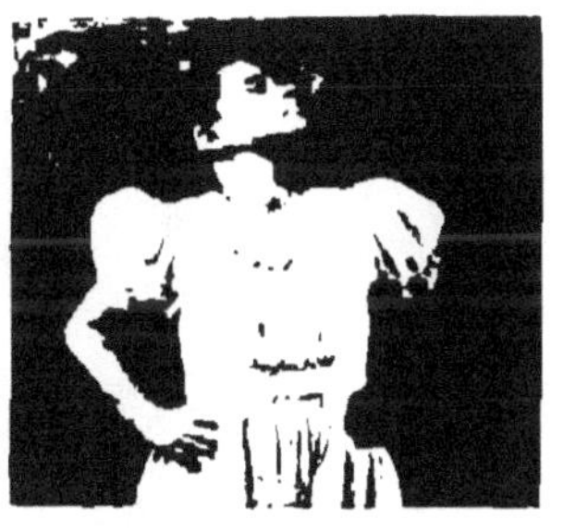

XLVIII.

On alternate days, same movement from foot backward-outward place.

HEAD MOVEMENT.—Standing or sitting; hips firm; head twist; from this position, *head backward bend.* (3–8 repetitions.) Direct this movement back of the head, not of the body. Take care that head is not inclined to side.

Massage as before prescribed.

CHEST MOVEMENT.—As previous prescription; hips firm; *head and upper spine backward bend.* (8 repetitions.)

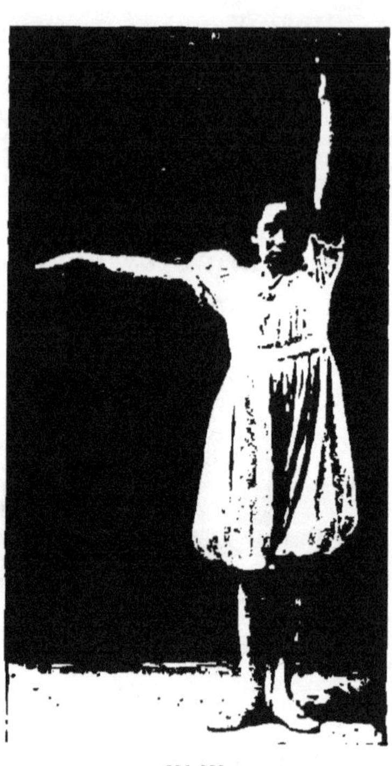

XLIX.

Massage for chest.

SHOULDER-BLADE MOVEMENT.—Arms upward bend; *left arm upward, right arm sideways, stretch simultaneously.* (5–8 repetitions.) Alternate at each repetition; *i. e.,* left arm sideways, right arm upward stretch.

Observe advice given in previous lessons regarding accuracy of movement and of posture.

The arm stretchings forward and backward

are valuable movements, but are not included in these lessons on account of the tendency to incorrect posture of head, chest, and abdomen during the practice.

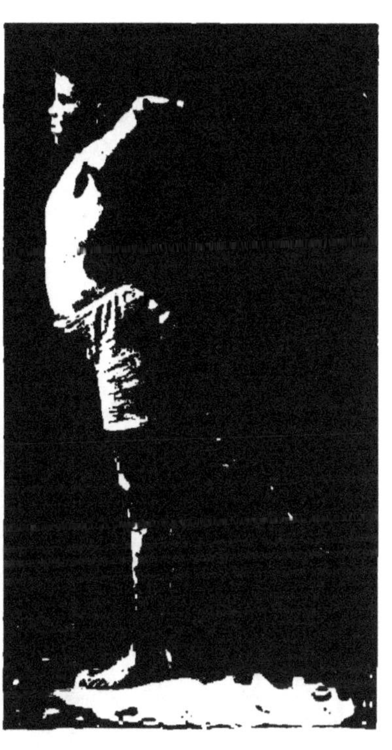

L.

Massage for arms or for finger-joints follows the shoulder-blade movements.

BALANCE MOVEMENT.—Hips firm; *leg backward stretch;* hold posture until good balance is attained; avoid wrong posture of foot; then *foot replace* to fundamental position. (3–8 repetitions.) In the backward stretch take care that the knee and ankle are fully extended, and that good chest and trunk posture is maintained. After good poise has been attained from hips firm position of hands, practice the same movement, holding arms in plane of shoulders (posture L.). The next step in progression is neck firm, and then the same movement from arms stretched upward. Make the movement more vigorous by *heel raise* from the balance position. This is the conventionalized "flying Mercury."

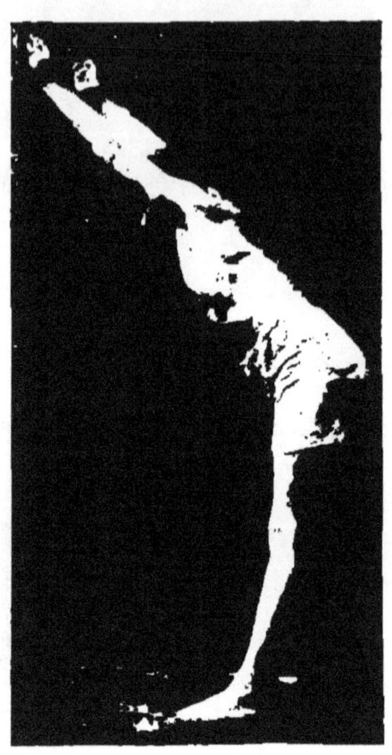

LI.

BACK MOVEMENT.—Stride-standing, or stride-sitting; arms upward bend (posture XXIV., lesson I.); trunk forward bend; *arms stretch in line with trunk.* (5–12 repetitions.)

The value of this movement and the cautions to be observed are obvious.

Increase the bend posture in accordance with flexibility of leg and thigh muscles.

Massage for back follows.

ABDOMINAL MOVEMENT.—Recumbent posture; hips firm (neck firm at discretion); *leg raise* (posture XXVII., lesson I.); *knee bend* (posture LII.); *knee stretch* (posture XXVIII., lesson I.); *leg downward sink.* (3–8 repetitions each.) See that the changes of the leg position are slow, and that a momentary pause is made between them. The foot must maintain

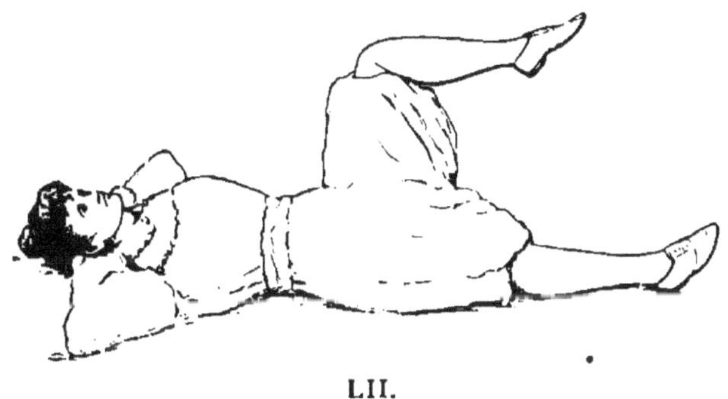

LII.

the ninety degrees angle required in standing. The movement begins with foot extension, consequently the energy is directed there. Manipulations for stomach and liver follow.

LATERAL TRUNK MOVEMENT.—Stride-sitting; neck firm; feet fixed; trunk twist; and from that position *trunk bend.* (5–8 repetitions from each side twist.) Complete the bend movements from the one side before assuming the twist position for the other. This is described in the preceding prescription. It may now be practiced standing, taking care that no twisting of hips is allowed.

Manipulations for colon, as directed in prescription I., follow.

LEG MOVEMENT.—Neck firm; stride-standing; *heels raise; knees bend;* hold posture a few moments; *knees stretch; heels sink.* (3–10 repetitions.) Movement described in previous prescription. Do not attempt this in case of pelvic weakness or hemorrhoidal tendency.

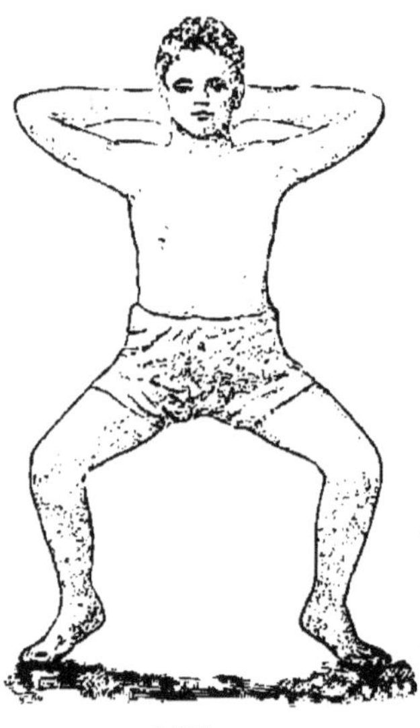

LIII.

RESPIRATORY MOVEMENT.—Arms *forward-upward raise, inhaling* (posture XLII., prescription I.); *sideways; hands turn at shoulder height* (posture LIV.); *downward sink, exhaling.* (10 repetitions.) Take care that head does not push forward.

Continue this prescription several weeks, possibly months, before beginning the following more vigorous one. I would recommend that these first two prescriptions be continued three months each—longer, if necessary for good

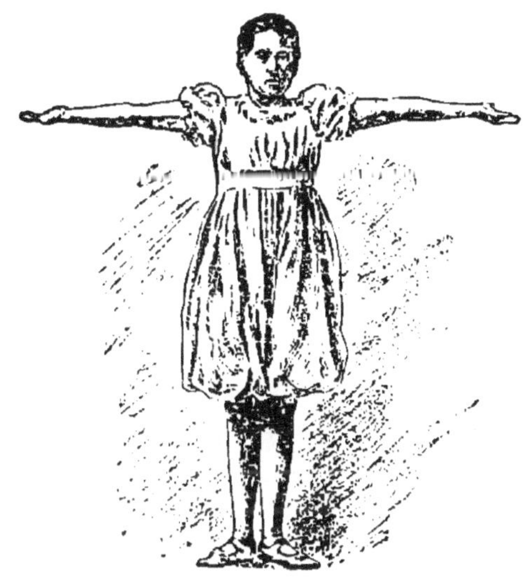

LIV.

muscular control—and that the following one be continued indefinitely.

MEMORANDUM OF PRESCRIPTION II

ADULTS

RESPIRATORY MOVEMENT.—*Arms sideways raise, inhaling.* (10 repetitions.)

FOOT MOVEMENT.—Neck firm; *foot outward place; heels raise;* hold; *heels sink; foot replace.* (5 repetitions.)

HEAD MOVEMENT.—Standing or sitting; hips firm; head twist and *backward bend.* (3–8 repetitions.)

CHEST MOVEMENT.—Standing; hips firm; *head and upper spine backward bend.* (8 repetitions.)

SHOULDER-BLADE MOVEMENT.—*Left arm upward, right arm sideways stretch, alternating.* (5–8 repetitions.)

BALANCE MOVEMENT.—Hips firm; arms raised sideways; neck firm; and arms stretched upward, in progression; *leg backward stretch.* (3–8 repetitions.) Later, same, *heel raise.*

BACK MOVEMENT.—Stride-standing or stride-sitting; arms upward bend; trunk forward bend; *arms stretch in line with trunk.* (5–12 repetitions.)

ABDOMINAL MOVEMENT.—Lying; neck firm or hips firm; *leg raise; knee bend; stretch; leg downward sink.* (3–8 repetitions.)

LATERAL TRUNK MOVEMENT.—Stride-sitting; neck firm; feet fixed; trunk twist; and from that position, *bend.* (5–8 repetitions.)

LEG MOVEMENT.—Neck firm; stride-standing; *heels raise; knees bend;* hold; *knees stretch; heels sink.* (3–10 repetitions.)

RESPIRATORY MOVEMENT.—*Arms forward-upward raise, inhaling; sideways-downward sink, exhaling.* (10 repetitions.)

CHAPTER XIV

PRESCRIPTIONS OF EXERCISE FOR HOME PRACTICE (*Continued*)

"For life is not to live, but to be well."—STERNE.

PRESCRIPTION III.—ADULTS. MORE VIGOROUS THAN THE PRECEDING

RESPIRATORY MOVEMENT.—*Arms sideways raise, inhaling*, as in prescription II. (10 repetitions.)

FOOT MOVEMENT.—From prescriptions I. and II., on alternate days; *i. e., foot forward* and *backward place, and heels raise*; and *outward* and *backward-outward, and heels raise.* (5 repetitions.) Use care in regard to posture and carriage.

HEAD MOVEMENT.—From prescriptions I. and II., on alternate days; *i. e.*, head twist, and *to the side bend*; and twist, and *backward bend.* (8 repetitions.)

Or, *head circumduction.* (5–8 repetitions each side.) Allow the head to move slowly and steadily around on the spine, using energy in only the muscles that control the movement, resisting it slightly.

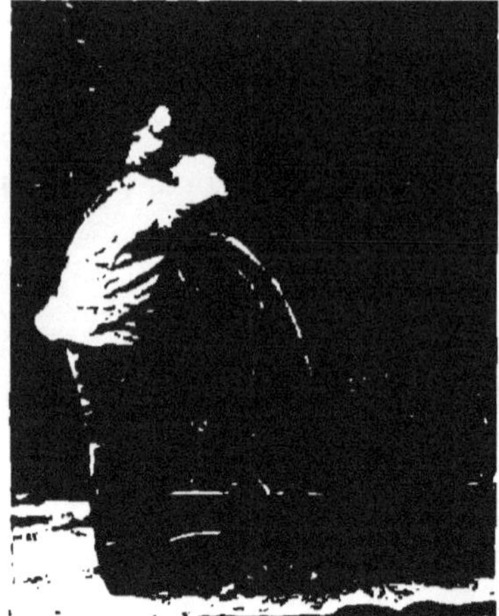

LV.

CHEST MOVEMENT.—Stride-standing; neck firm; *head and upper spine backward bend.* (5–8 repetitions.) Observe cautions for good chest posture.

Or, stride-kneeling against shoulder pressure, to insure good position of spine at waist; from this posture practice the *chest raise.* (3 8 repetitions.)

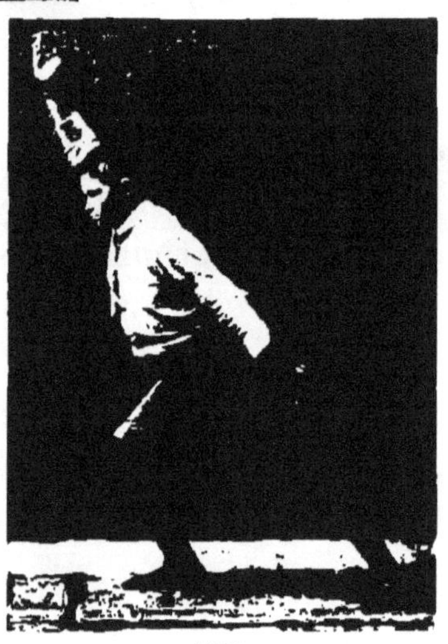

LVI.

SHOULDER-BLADE MOVEMENT.—Arms upward bend; *right arm*

upward, and left arm backward stretch, and right forward fall-out. (3-8 repetitions each.) The fall-out means a long step with forward knee bent, backward leg to be held in tense position. Use care that the arm-stretch and fall-out are made simultaneously; that hand is

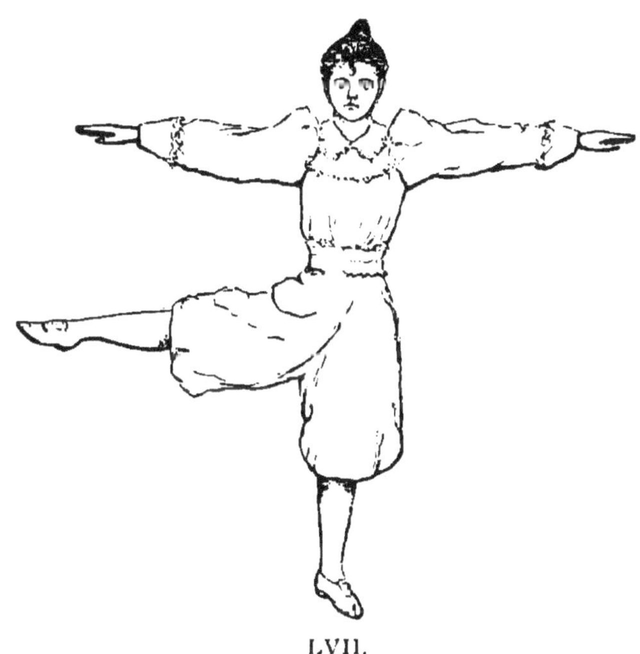

LVII.

in line with arm, and that extended leg and back are in line.

BALANCE MOVEMENT.—Neck firm, or arms raised sideways; *extend foot, and raise leg side-*

ways. (5–8 repetitions.) The movement must be executed slowly, else balance cannot be

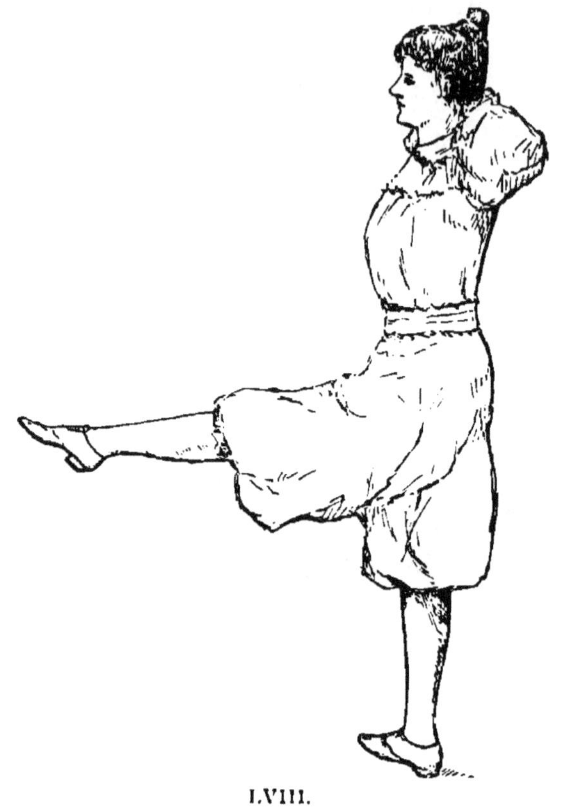

LVIII.

attained. Begin by raising the foot but slightly, and patiently continue, approaching the angle of posture LVII. as flexibility permits.

Or, *leg forward raise* (posture LVIII.). (5–8 repetitions.) Take care to maintain good chest posture.

BACK MOVEMENT.—Stride-standing; arms stretched upward; trunk forward bend; *arm parting*. (8–12 repetitions.)

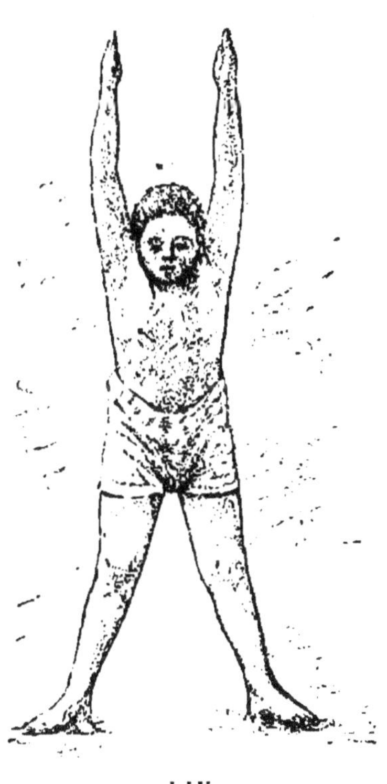

LIX.

Assume posture LIX. as directed, and lower the arms resistively to shoulder height (the same as posture LIV.), and raise them resistively to former position.

Or, in later practice, stride-standing; arms stretch upward; *trunk forward-downward bend*. (3–8 repetitions.)

Do not attempt this until muscles are properly trained and conditions are favorable.

ABDOMINAL MOVEMENT.—Recumbent posture; hips firm; *extend ankles, and raise legs* simultaneously. (3–8 repetitions.)

The early practice should be merely an attempt at raising the legs simultaneously, directing the energy to the feet. Continue this patiently for days, and gradually the muscles

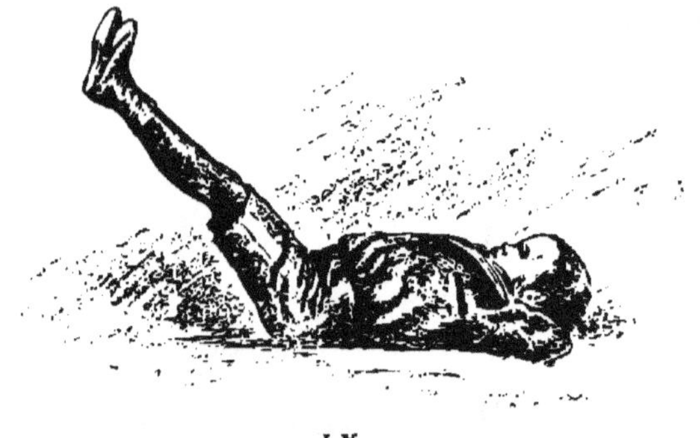

LX.

will obey the mind in the more complete execution of the movement. It must be a slow, steady pull with the extensor muscles, and the relaxing must also be gradual, never a *dropping*. Breathe freely.

Later, the same movement may be practiced from neck firm position. (3–8 repetitions.) Properly approached and executed, it is a most valuable exercise for strengthening the abdominal walls, consequently, the organs; indiscriminately practiced, it is one of the most harmful.

A more vigorous movement, one that follows this in progression, is *legs circumduction.* (3–8 repetitions.) The legs are raised, and simultaneously carried in the same direction, the movement being from the hips. These vigorous movements are more advantageously practiced if an attendant holds the elbows

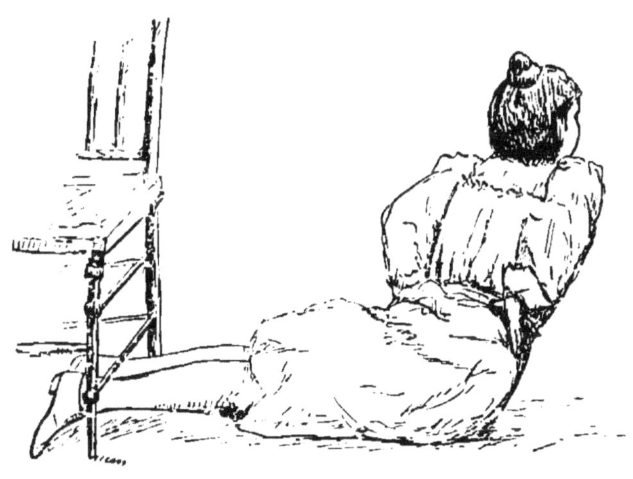

LXI.

down, as the energy is the better localized when leverage is thus aided.

LATERAL TRUNK MOVEMENT. — Chest-lying; feet fixed; hips firm; *trunk raise, and bend.* (2–8 repetitions for each side.) It is best that normal chest-lying position is assumed between each succession of two repetitions, for a few moments' rest.

Observe cautions previously mentioned in regard to raising the trunk.

After a few weeks' practice, the same movement may possibly be taken from neck firm position. (2–8 repetitions.) This, however, should not be undertaken, except under most favorable conditions.

Jump Movement. — From toe-knee-bend position, heels raise, knees bend (posture XLVII., prescription I.), *jump*, straightening the legs in the jump, and landing in same toe-knee-bend position; hold balance until good poise is attained; then *knees stretch, heels sink*, as usual. (3–5 repetitions.)

Practice also a jump *forward, outward*, and *sideways*; also *jump down from slight elevation*, as foot-stool, etc., using always the same cautions regarding the preparatory movement and the landing.

These jump movements are invaluable in training to good poise. They also increase circulation, consequently greater demands are made on heart action and respiratory organs. These organs, however, should not be taxed sufficiently to cause discomfort.

SLOW LEG MOVEMENT.—Neck firm; *heels raise.* (10 repetitions.)

RESPIRATORY MOVEMENT.—As prescription II., adding alternate trunk twist; *i. e.*, on the forward-upward raise of arms, *twist to side;* on the sideways-downward sink, *twist to front.* (10 repetitions.)

MEMORANDUM OF PRESCRIPTION III

ADULTS

RESPIRATORY MOVEMENT.—*Arms sideways raise, inhaling.* (10 repetitions.)

FOOT MOVEMENT.—*Foot place forward;* also *backward*, and *heels raise.* (5 repetitions.) On alternate days, *foot outward;* also *backward-outward place*, and *heels raise.* (5 repetitions.)

HEAD MOVEMENT.—Head twist, and to the *side bend.* (8 repetitions.) On alternate days, twist and *backward bend.* (8 repetitions.)

CHEST MOVEMENT.— Stride-standing or stride-kneeling against shoulder pressure; neck firm; *head and upper spine backward bend.* (5–8 repetitions.)

SHOULDER-BLADE MOVEMENT.—Arms upward bend; *right arm upward, left arm backward stretch, and right forward fall-out;* alternate with left side. (3–8 repetitions.)

BALANCE MOVEMENT.—Neck firm, or arms raised sideways; *leg sideways raise.* (5–8 repetitions.)

Or, *leg forward raise.* (5–8 repetitions.)

BACK MOVEMENT.—Stride-standing; arms upward stretch; trunk forward bend; *arm parting.* (8–12 repetitions.)

Or, from stride-stretch posture, trunk forward-downward bend. (3–8 repetitions.)

ABDOMINAL MOVEMENT.—Lying; hips firm or neck firm; *legs raise.* (3–8 repetitions.) Later, *legs circumduction.* (3–8 repetitions.)

LATERAL TRUNK MOVEMENT.—Chest lying; feet fixed; *trunk raise* and *bend.* (2–8 repetitions.)

JUMP MOVEMENT.—From toe-knee-bend position, *jump*, landing in same position. (3–5 repetitions.)

SLOW LEG MOVEMENT.—Neck firm; *heels raise*. (10 repetitions.)

RESPIRATORY MOVEMENT.—*Arms forward-upward raise, and trunk to side twist, inhaling; arms sideways-downward sink, and trunk to front twist, inhaling*. (10 repetitions.)

Continue the massage, if necessary.

It must be remembered that this prescription represents very vigorous work, and should not be attempted until preparatory exercise has been long continued.

CHAPTER XV

SWEDISH MOVEMENTS FROM RECUMBENT POSTURE, FOR ADULTS

"Our foster-nurse of nature is repose."—SHAKSPEARE.

THIS prescription of exercise is arranged for days of especial fatigue, or on recuperation from illness, or when any causes are present that render it necessary to discontinue exercise of a more vigorous character. The postures assumed for practice or for rest are as follows: *Lying* (if a pillow is necessary, it should extend under shoulders as well as the head, to give advantage in respiration and in chest posture). *Half-lying* (posture LXII.); the body should be at an angle of about forty-five degrees with the legs, and the back should be firmly supported, as with a bed-rest, folding table, inverted chair, etc. *Hook-lying* (posture LXIV.); the legs and thighs are at an angle of about forty-five degrees. *Sit-lying* (see posture XCIV., chapter XXIII., on Regulation of Flesh); the knees are bent over the side of a couch. *Chest-lying* (explained in previous chapters); *knee-chest* (posture LXVII.). In this posture it is often best to bend over a small hair pillow, for the purpose of giving good support to abdominal viscera.

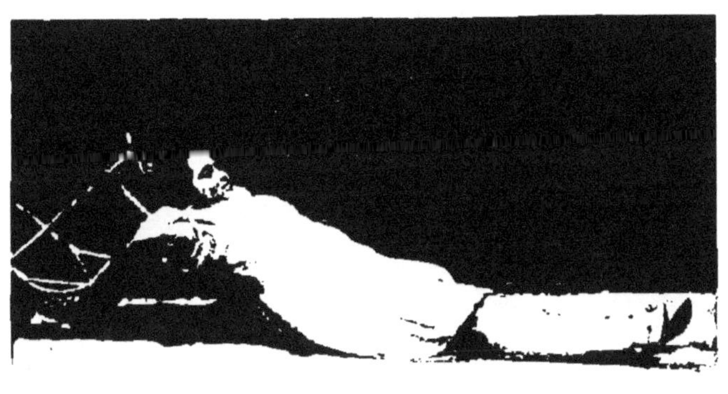

LXII.—HALF-LYING.

Half-lying is preferable to *lying*, in case of tendency to excess of blood to brain. *Half-lying* or *hook-lying* is preferable to *lying*, in early practice, in case of especially weak abdominal walls.

In cases of pelvic weakness, the physician should decide posture for movements. (See chapter on Diagnosis.)

The movements should be practiced upon the floor, or a hard couch, in preference to a soft couch, which yields too readily to the form.

Practice the movements slowly.

Respiratory Movement. — Lying, half-lying, or hook-lying; neck firm; *deep breathing.* (10 repetitions.)

Or, from either posture, arms upward bend; *elbows raise, inhaling; sink, exhaling.* (10 repetitions.) (See postures XXIV. and XXV., lesson I.)

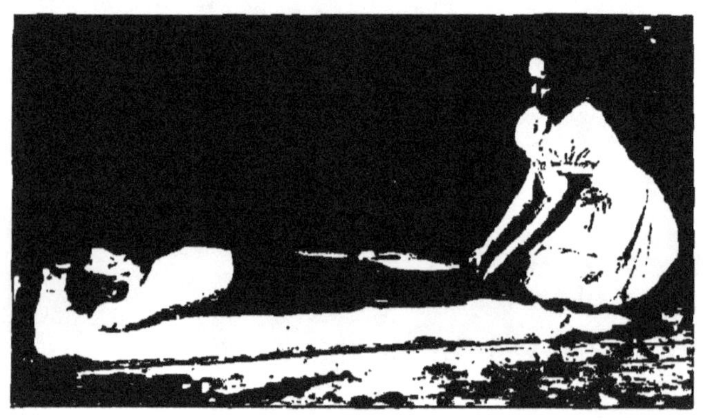

LXIII.

Foot Movement. — Lying or half-lying; hips firm or neck firm; *bend and stretch ankles* resistively. (10-20 repetitions.) (See fifth movement described in lesson III.) More advantage is gained from practice of this movement if applied resistance is given (posture LXIII.). The attendant places her hands on the patient's insteps, and resists the patient's ankle bend, and changes position of hands, pressing against the balls of the feet, to resist the ankle stretch. The change of hand position should be made without any decided pause in the resistive force, if possible. The resistance is light or heavy, in accordance with patient's strength.

SHOULDER-BLADE MOVEMENT. — Lying, half-lying, or hook-lying; arms at side, or raised in line with shoulders; *arm rotation.* (10–20 repetitions.) Fourth movement described in lesson I.

Hand extension, both hands simultaneously, should follow this. (8–10 repetitions.) The energy is directed to the finger-tips, and the movement includes the contraction of all the muscles on the back of the fingers and hand. Isolate all other muscles. Do not make this a wrist movement.

This and the foot movement are invaluable in directing the blood current to the extremities, and thus inducing repose. Alternating these (20 repetitions each), followed by the respiratory movement before described, will frequently induce sleep for those mentally over-burdened, by directing the blood current to the extremities, and thus relieving the over-charged brain.

CHEST MOVEMENT.—Lying, half-lying, or hook-lying; arms upward bend (posture XXIV., lesson I.); *arm extension in line with trunk, resistively.* (5–12 repetitions.)

Or, from either posture, *arm pulling* by an attendant (posture LXIX., chapter XVI.). (3–8 repetitions). The attendant must make the movement a steady, slow one, the patient resisting slightly so as to employ well the muscles used in chest raising. Increase this resistance at discretion. Breathe freely, but do not make it a respiratory movement; *i. e.*, do not force the muscles of respiration, nor make the breathing rhythmic with the movement. The advisability of this movement must be decided by the patient's condition. If it is not wise to extend her arms over her head, omit the movement.

FOOT MOVEMENT.—Repeat the one described above, or substitute for it *foot circumduction*, described in lesson III. (8–20 repetitions.)

Or, *foot parting.* (8–20 repetitions.) Bring the toes in touch, closing the usual angle of the feet, and resistively resume the angle. Much advantage is gained from applied resistance, the attendant pressing her hands on outer side of patient's feet, and resisting the movement in accordance with patient's strength. This movement improves the muscles that rotate the thigh; the energy, however, must be directed to the extremities.

BACK MOVEMENT.—Chest-lying; hips firm; feet fixed; *head and shoulders raise* (posture XXXV., lesson III.). (3–8 repetitions.)

Or, from same position, *arms stretch sideways* (posture XLV., prescription I.); observe carefully the descriptions and the cautions.

ABDOMINAL MOVEMENT. — Lying; neck firm; hips firm in case of weak abdominal walls; *leg raise* (posture XXVII., lesson I.). (3–8 repetitions.)

Or, from same posture, *leg circumduction*, described in seventh movement, lesson III. (3–8 repetitions.)

Or, in case of prolapsed condition of pelvic organs, or extreme fatigue from standing or walking, assume hook-lying posture; neck firm; *raise hips slowly*, until the trunk is in line with knees and shoulders; hold the posture during one or two deep breathings, as the lowering and raising of the diaphragm from

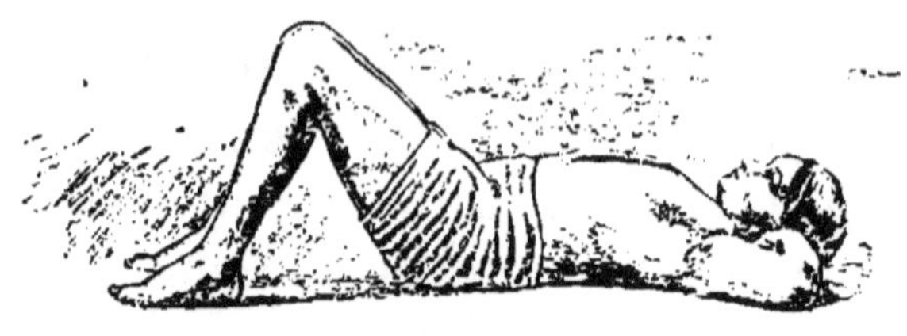

LXIV.

this position is valuable involuntary massage for internal organs, and helps greatly in restoring their normal position, and strengthening

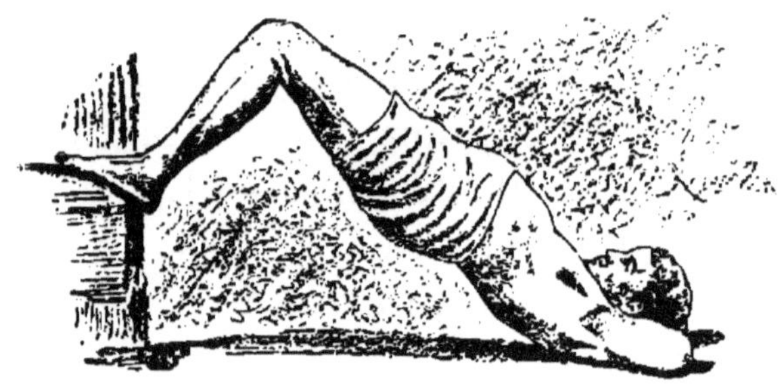

LXV.

their muscles of support. Lower the trunk slowly to former position. (3–8 repetitions.)

After a few weeks' practice, the hook-lying

position may be made by placing the feet on a couch, and executing the movement as posture LXV.

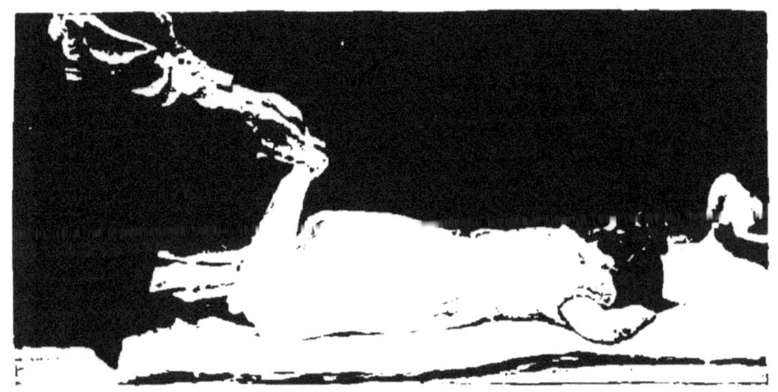

LXVI.

In the cases of pelvic weakness that demand chest-lying position instead of these described,

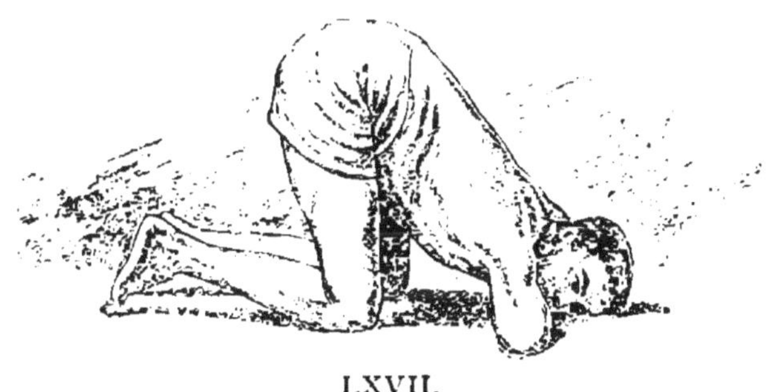

LXVII.

posture LXVI. is recommended. From chest-lying position, the patient will bend knees, and *extend them resistively.* (5–12 repetitions.) Applied resistance on the extensor movement, as shown in the picture, is of great advantage.

In place of this movement, posture LXVII.

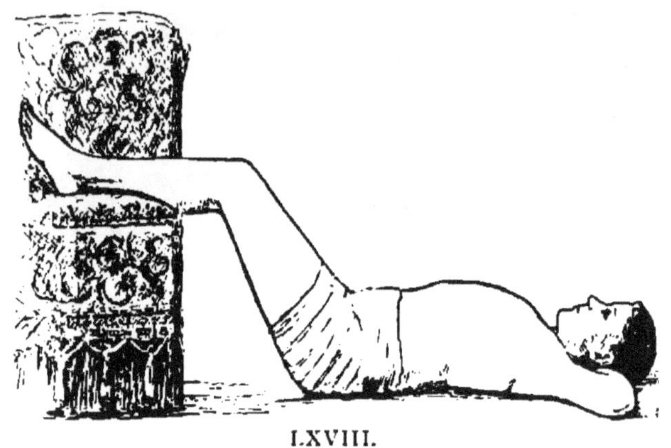

LXVIII.

is often recommended. The influence of this is obvious.

LATERAL TRUNK MOVEMENT.—Lying; neck firm; *direct the energy to intercostals, and transverse muscles of abdomen, as if to turn on the side; hold the muscles energized during a few heart-beats, and gradually relax them.* No effort should be made with the limbs. (3–8 repetitions.)

Or, from hook-lying posture, hips raise, and *alternately twist the trunk.* (2–5 repetitions.)

Resume former position for a few moments' rest, and repeat the movement.

In case patient's conditions demand chest-lying posture, employ very mildly the lateral trunk movement described in chapter XVI., posture LXXIII.

These three specific movements should be omitted on days when nature demands rest instead of exercise. When practiced, a few minutes' rest should be taken between the sets of movements from posture LXIV., LXVII., LXVIII.

Or, chest-lying; with one knee drawn up to relax the stretch on abdominal walls.

FOOT MOVEMENT.—Repeat either of those described above.

RESPIRATORY MOVEMENT.—Repeat either of those described above.

Massage and manipulations for weak tissues should follow movements that energize those muscles. (See chapter on Massage.)

MEMORANDUM OF RECUMBENT POSTURE MOVEMENTS

ADULTS

RESPIRATORY MOVEMENT.—Lying, half-lying, or hook-lying; neck firm; *deep breathing.* (10 repetitions.)

Or, arms upward bend; *elbows raise; inhaling.* (10 repetitions.)

FOOT MOVEMENT.—Lying or half-lying; hips firm or neck firm; *bend and stretch ankles.* (10–20 repetitions.)

SHOULDER-BLADE MOVEMENT. — Lying, half-lying, or hook-lying; arms at side, or in line with shoulders; *arm rotation.* (10–20 repetitions.)

Hand extension. (8–20 repetitions.)

CHEST MOVEMENT.—Lying, half-lying, or hook-lying; arms upward bend (posture XXIV., Lesson I.); *arm extension in line with trunk, resistively.* (5–12 repetitions.)

Or, *arm pulling.* (3–8 repetitions.)

FOOT MOVEMENT.—Lying or half-lying; *bend and stretch ankles.* (10–20 repetitions.)

Or, *foot circumduction.* (8–10 repetitions.)

Or, *foot parting.* (8–20 repetitions.)

BACK MOVEMENT.—Chest-lying; hips firm; feet fixed; *head and shoulders raise.* (3–8 repetitions.)

ABDOMINAL MOVEMENT.—Lying; neck firm or hips firm; *leg raise.* (8 repetitions.)

Or, *leg circumduction.* (8 repetitions.)

Or, hook-lying; *hips raise.* (3–8 repetitions.)

Or, chest-lying; knees bend; *extend resistively.* (5–12 repetitions.)

Or, knee-chest posture; *rest.*

Lateral Trunk Movement.—Lying; neck firm; *energize the muscles used in the trunk twist.* (3–8 repetitions.)

Or, hook-lying; hips raise; *trunk twist.* (2–5 repetitions.)

Foot Movement.—Repeat either of those described above.

Respiratory Movement.—Repeat either of those described above.

Massage to follow movements if necessary.

CHAPTER XVI

PRESCRIPTIONS OF EXERCISE FOR CHILDREN'S HOME PRACTICE

"Children are travellers newly arrived in a strange country; we should, therefore, make conscience not to mislead them."—LOCKE.

PRESCRIPTION I.—RECUMBENT POSTURE MOVEMENTS

MOVEMENTS used in the foregoing lessons will be employed, and should be well studied before directing these for children, as the descriptions are more in detail. Accuracy must be observed.

Symmetry of growth, firmness and flexibility of muscle, and health of organs is the aim with children.

Take care that movements are not jerkily or rapidly practiced. The influence of such on nerve strength is unfavorable, especially with children of nervous temperament.

This prescription of movements, mainly from recumbent postures, precedes the one from standing postures, as it insures good position of spine, and enables the child to localize the energy to the groups of muscles employed, which is less easily accomplished if his mind is also on posture. Following this is one from standing postures, of corresponding character as regards amount of energy involved.

The two prescriptions may be alternated with good results, preventing the child from tiring of either, although I recommend that a few weeks' practice be first given the recumbent.

These may be continued indefinitely, and the two that follow, in chapters XVIII. and XIX., may be begun at discretion. Massage may be used as directed in lessons for adults. This is of great value with growing children. It helps especially the circulation and nerve current, and aids in establishing good digestive power.

RESPIRATORY MOVEMENT. — Lying; half-

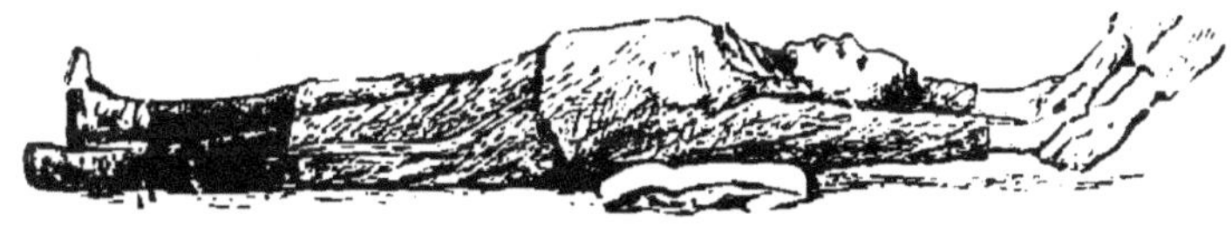

LXIX.

lying, if preferable; arms upward bend; *arm extension in line with trunk, inhaling.* Described as chest movement in Recumbent Postures. (10 repetitions.)

Or, *arm pulling in line with trunk* (posture LXIX.).

Foot Movement.—Lying; neck firm; *bend and stretch ankles.* (10 repetitions.) The movement must be slow and resistive. With young or delicate children it is best to have applied resistance. (See description, and posture LXIII. recumbent posture lesson.) This is excellent practice for children who are "pigeon-toed;" care must be taken to maintain foot angle of ninety degrees. It is recumbent walking, really, and forces the circulation in the extremities without taxing spinal muscles, as in poising the body. It rests the body by drawing blood to lower muscles.

Chest Raising.—Chest-lying; feet fixed; *i. e.*, placed under a piece of heavy furniture, or held firmly by attendant; hips firm; head and shoulders raise; *head rotation*, including both to the left and the right side. (2 repetitions.) Relax the spinal muscles, and rest in former position a few moments; then raise the head and shoulders, and execute two repetitions again. Described in back movement, lesson III., adults. Take care that the face is raised in plane of the wall, and that the movement is slow, not jerky. This movement is a valuable one if properly practiced. Holding the trunk suspended by the long muscles of the spine

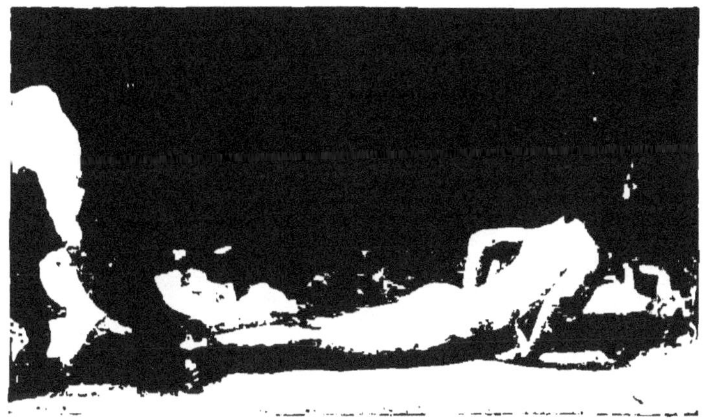

LXX.

while the muscles of the upper spine are exercised, cannot fail to correct droop posture of head and lax condition of shoulders.

FOOT MOVEMENT.—As already described in this lesson. This is repeated here to draw the blood to the lower extremities, after practice of the chest movement. It may be omitted with robust children, if time is limited.

BACK MOVEMENT.—Chest-lying; feet fixed;

arms upward bend; head and shoulders raise; *arm extension sideways, resistively.* (3–5 repetitions.) Slowly relax the muscles; those that control the lower spine first, then the shoulders, and lastly those that control the head, and rest a few moments; then raise trunk, and repeat the movement again. (3–5 repetitions.)

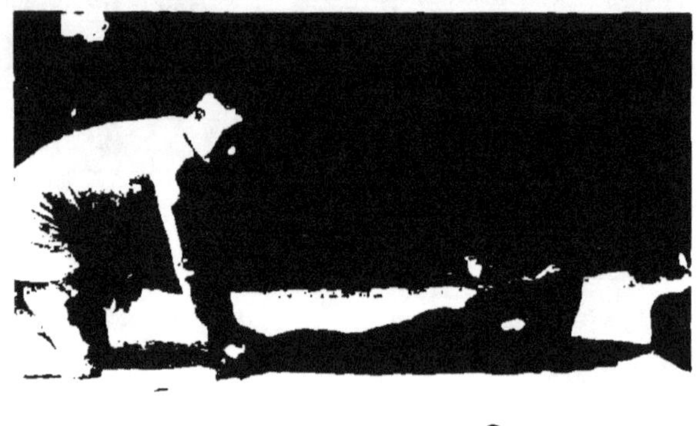

LXXI.

Be sure that arm extension is complete, and that the face is raised so that the muscles of the upper spine are well used. Hold arm extension a few heart-beats before bending the arms again. Breathe freely. Increase the work by adding another group of repetitions, as, 3 repetitions, rest; 3 repetitions, rest; 3 repetitions, rest.

ABDOMINAL MOVEMENT. — Lying; neck firm; *leg raise.* (8 repetitions each.) Observe directions given in lesson I. for adults.

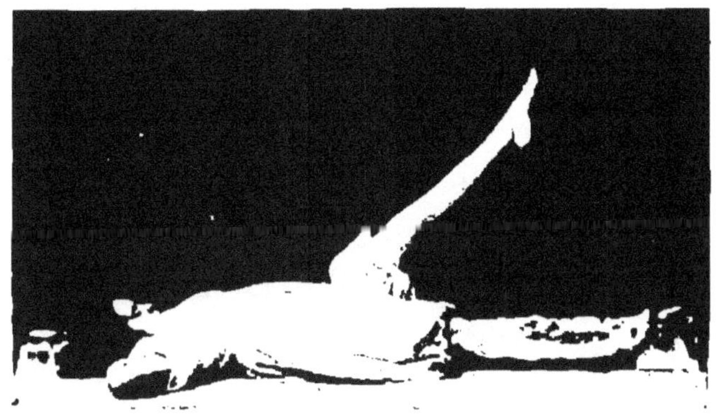

LXXII.

Or, *leg circumduction.* Described in lesson III. for adults. (5-8 repetitions).

Or, lying; neck firm; *leg raise; knee bend* to angle of ninety degrees, foot extended; *knee stretch; leg sink.* (Posture LII., chapter XIII.) (3-8 repetitions.) Observe accuracy in this; a pause should occur between the different postures of the movement. This movement should not be omitted, especially with girls. It must, however, be practiced discreetly; the energy increased gradually, not forced. Great advantage to health of internal organs and to symmetry of the figure, in preventing lax condition of abdominal walls, will follow exercise of these muscles.

LATERAL TRUNK MOVEMENT.—Chest-lying: feet fixed; hips firm; head and shoulders raise; *trunk bend; i. e.*, carry to side; resume simple chest-lying position of trunk, and relax muscles for rest position. (3–8 repetitions each side.) Take care that child does not hold the breath, and that the movement is not rapid.

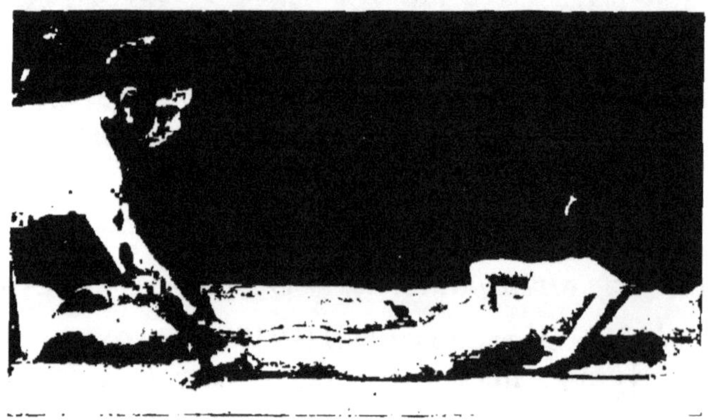

LXXIII.

FOOT MOVEMENT.—As already described in this lesson.

RESPIRATORY MOVEMENT.—As already described in this lesson.

MEMORANDUM OF RECUMBENT POSTURE MOVEMENTS, PRESCRIPTION I

CHILDREN

RESPIRATORY MOVEMENT.—Lying; arms upward bend; *arm extension* or *arm pulling in line with trunk.* (10 repetitions.)

FOOT MOVEMENT.—Lying; neck firm; *bend and stretch ankles.* (10 repetitions.)

CHEST RAISING.—Chest-lying; feet fixed; head and shoulders raise; *head rotation.* (2 repetitions, rest; 2 repetitions, rest.)

FOOT MOVEMENT.—Repeat one mentioned above.

BACK MOVEMENT.—Chest-lying; feet fixed; arms upward bend; head and shoulders raise; *arm extension sideways.* (3 repetitions, rest; 3 repetitions, rest; increase at discretion to 5.)

ABDOMINAL MOVEMENT.—Lying; neck firm; *leg raise.* (S repetitions.)

Or, *leg circumduction.* (5 repetitions.)

Or, *leg raise; knee bend; stretch; downward sink.* (S repetitions.)

LATERAL TRUNK MOVEMENT.—Chest-lying; feet fixed; hips firm; head and shoulders raise; *trunk bend to side.* (3–S repetitions.)

FOOT MOVEMENT.—Repeat the one mentioned above.

RESPIRATORY MOVEMENT.—Repeat the one mentioned above.

CHAPTER XVII

PRESCRIPTIONS FOR CHILDREN (*Continued*).

"Childhood shows the man as morning shows the day."—MILTON.

PRESCRIPTION I.—EXERCISE FROM STANDING POSTURE FOR CHILDREN. TO ALTERNATE WITH, OR USE IN PLACE OF, THE PRECEDING

THE chest, shoulder-blade, and balance movements are especially important for children. (See definitions of movements, chapter VIII.)

RESPIRATORY MOVEMENT.—Stride-standing; *arms sideways raise, inhaling; downward sink, exhaling.* (10 repetitions.)

HEAD MOVEMENT.—*Head sideways bend.* (8 repetitions.) Described in lesson II. for adults.

CHEST MOVEMENT.—Stride-standing; neck firm; *head and upper spine backward bend.* (5 8 repetitions.) As described in prescription III. for adults. Do not attempt this unless good posture is maintained; the arch should be made with the upper spine; tipping backward from the waist must be carefully avoided. Breathe freely, but not in rhythm with the movement.

SHOULDER-BLADE MOVEMENT.—Arm

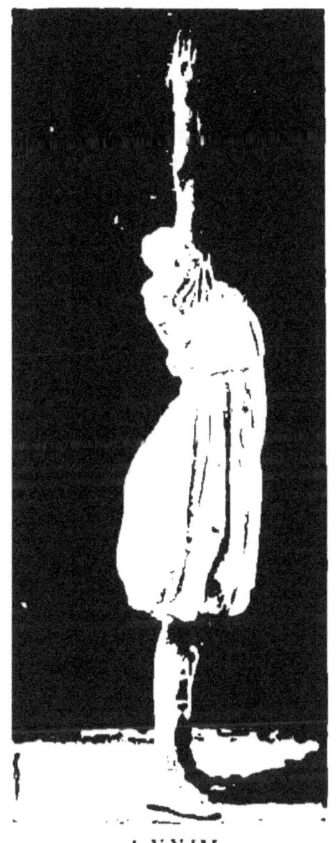

LXXIV.

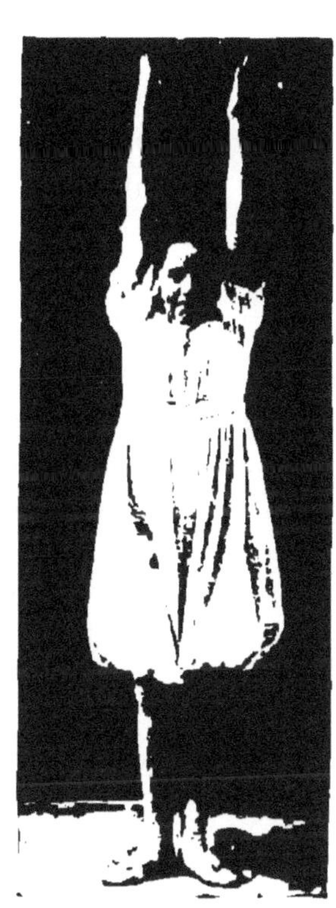

LXXV.

stretching as described in prescription I. for adults; *i. e., arms bend and sideways stretch;*

bend and upward stretch; bend and downward stretch. (3-5 repetitions.) Be careful to keep good chest posture, to make arm stretching slow and resistive, and aim to reach a point beyond the possible stretch. The great value of the movement lies in the enforced extension. Direct the thought to the finger-tips. The forward and backward stretchings are omitted on account of liability to wrong position of shoulder-blades and chest in executing the movement.

BALANCE MOVEMENT.—Neck firm; heels raise; *slowly walk forward on toes.* (10-20 steps.)

Place a book or other easily movable object on the head, to insure steady carriage. Hold each step until balance is perfectly controlled. Maintain correct posture of toes; *i. e.*, angle of ninety degrees, in every foot placing.

It is also valuable balance practice to walk on a raised object, as a pole, representing a railroad track.

Practice walking on toes with eyes closed, and observe whether or not straight direction is possible.

Practice also slow walk backward on toes, pausing between steps to attain good poise.

Practice all these from different arm postures; *i. e.*, hips firm; neck firm; arms raised sideways; and, later, arms extended upward; observing accurate position of head, arms, and chest in all.

Balance movements are invaluable in training the will power, and in training to muscular sense and coördination.

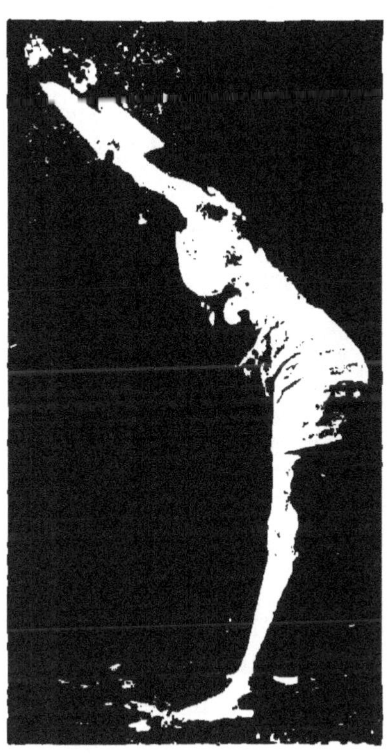

LXXVI.

BACK MOVEMENT.—Stride-standing; arms upward bend; trunk forward bend, from hips only; spinal column must be held in normal position; face raised; from this posture, *arm stretch in line with trunk.* (5–12 repetitions.)

Use care that the hands are shoulder width apart, that the head does not push forward, and that the arms are well raised.

In place of this, from horizontal bar, which can easily be adjusted in a doorway, suspend by the hands, and gradually raise the weight by flexing the elbows, keeping the face raised. (3–8 repetitions, resting between.)

LATERAL TRUNK MOVEMENT.—Neck firm; *side bend.* (8 repetitions each.) Described in lesson III., posture XXXVII., adults.

On alternate days, stride-sitting; *side twist.* (8 repetitions.) Described in lesson II., posture XXXII., adults. Observe the cautions mentioned there. Increase the bend as practice continues.

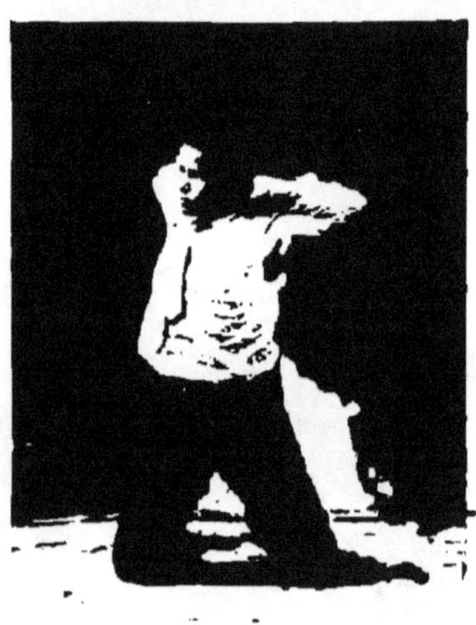

LXXVII.

Or, stride-kneeling; neck firm; *alternate trunk twist.* (5–8 repetitions.) The movement must involve energy; *i. e.*, after the normal limit of the twist is reached, force the energy. It is valuable for health of digestive apparatus, as well as for muscular control.

JUMP MOVEMENT.—*Heels raise; knees bend;* from this posture, *jump*, straightening the legs in the jump, and landing in toe-knee-bend posture; *i. e.*, heels raised; knees bent; hold the position until perfect balance is attained; then return to first posture; *i. e., knees stretch; heels sink.* (3-8 repetitions.) Described in prescription III., adults.

Progression in the jump is very interesting to children. After good poise is attained through practice, they may jump forward, outward, or sideways, as indicated by the foot chart, lesson II., adults. The next step in progression is to land, facing at angle of ninety degrees, and later, one hundred and eighty degrees, from start posture. Later, we combine the two; *i. e.*, the direction of jump, and the landing at different angle from that of the start.

SLOW LEG MOVEMENT.—Neck firm; *heels raise; heels sink.* (10 repetitions.)

This may be omitted unless the blood current has been forced too much by the jump exercise, and needs this to regulate it.

RESPIRATORY MOVEMENT.—*Arms sideways raise; hands turn* at shoulder height; *upward raise, inhaling; sideways sink; hands turn* at

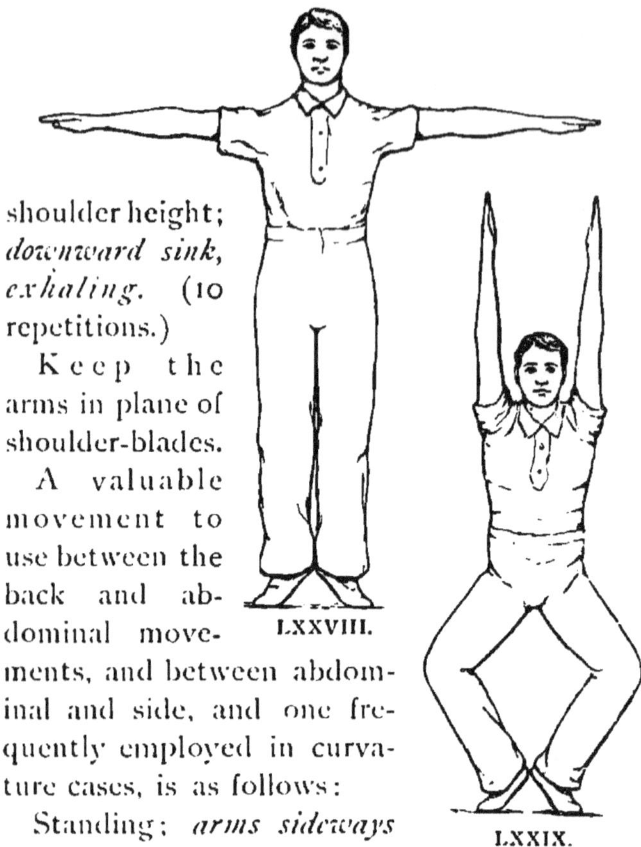

LXXVIII.

LXXIX.

shoulder height; *downward sink, exhaling.* (10 repetitions.)

Keep the arms in plane of shoulder-blades.

A valuable movement to use between the back and abdominal movements, and between abdominal and side, and one frequently employed in curvature cases, is as follows:

Standing; *arms sideways raise and heels raise* simultaneously (posture LXXVIII.); *hands turn and arms upward raise, and knees bend* simultaneously (posture LXXIX.); *arms sideways sink and knees stretch; hands turn and arms downward sink, and heels sink.* (3-8 repetitions.)

It brings excellent coördination of the entire muscular system, and may be used in addition to the other movements, as suggested, or in place of balance or jump movements.

After the practice has been continued long enough for good poise to be easily attained, it may be employed as a respiratory movement.

This movement may be used in the advanced work for adults.

MEMORANDUM OF PRESCRIPTION I—STANDING POSTURE

Children

Respiratory Movement.—*Arms sideways raise, inhaling.* (10 repetitions.)

Head Movement.—*Head sideways bend.* (8 repetitions.)

Chest Movement.—Stride-standing; neck firm; *head and upper spine backward bend.* (5–8 repetitions.)

Shoulder-blade Movement.—*Arms upward bend; sideways stretch; bend; upward stretch; bend; downward stretch.* (3–5 repetitions.)

Balance Movement.—Neck firm (balance book on head); *slowly walk forward on toes.*

Back Movement.—Stride-standing; arms upward bend; trunk forward bend; *arm extension in line with trunk.* (5–12 repetitions.)

Or, suspend from horizontal bar; *flex elbows.*

Lateral Trunk Movement.—Stride-sitting or stride-kneeling; neck firm; *side bend.* (8 repetitions.) On alternate days, *side twist.* (8 repetitions.)

Jump Movement.—*Heels raise; knees bend; jump; knees stretch; heels sink.* (3–8 repetitions.)

Slow Leg Movement.—Neck firm; *heels raise.* (10 repetitions.)

Respiratory Movement.—*Arms sideways-upward raise, inhaling; sideways-downward sink, exhaling.* (10 repetitions.)

(See definition of postures LXXVIII. and LXXIX.)

CHAPTER XVIII

PRESCRIPTIONS FOR CHILDREN (*Continued*)

"Health is every child's birthright."—ANON.

PRESCRIPTION II.—RECUMBENT POSTURE MOVEMENTS

RESPIRATORY MOVEMENT.—As corresponding movement from either of the previous prescriptions.

CHEST RAISING.—Chest-lying; feet fixed; arms upward bend; head and shoulders raise; *arm extension sideways.* (5 repetitions, rest; 5 repetitions, rest.) Described in back movement, prescription I., recumbent movements for children.

FOOT MOVEMENT.—Lying; neck firm; *foot parting, resistively; i. e.,* bring feet in close touch, and separate extremities again, resistively, to broad angle. (10 repetitions.) Described in recumbent posture lesson for adults.

BACK MOVEMENT.—Chest-lying; feet fixed; neck firm; *head and shoulders raise.* (3–8 repetitions.) Rest between repetitions. If this is too vigorous a posture, continue the practice from hips firm in place of neck firm position.

Or, chest-lying; feet fixed; arms upward

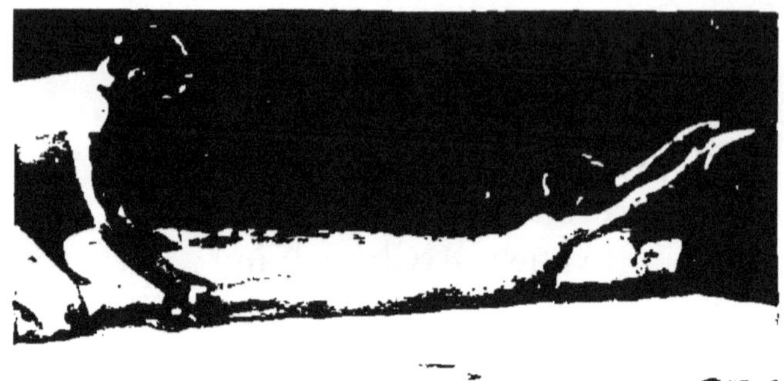

LXXX.

bend; head and shoulder raise; *arm pulling in line with trunk* (posture LXXX.). (2 repetitions, rest; 2 repetitions, rest; increase at discretion to 5 repetitions, rest; 5 repetitions, rest.)

Later, this may be practiced as *arm extension* without aid of additional attendant.

ABDOMINAL MOVEMENT. — Lying; neck firm; *legs raise* simultaneously. (3–8 repetitions.)

Begin by extending the feet, and only attempting to raise the legs. Subsequent practice will bring skill in making the movement complete. It must not be an impulse, but a slow raise, and equally slow return to rest posture. It is possible that full three months of practice will be necessary before an accurate *legs raise* to ninety degrees is attained. Use as much care with children as with adults in progressing the work.

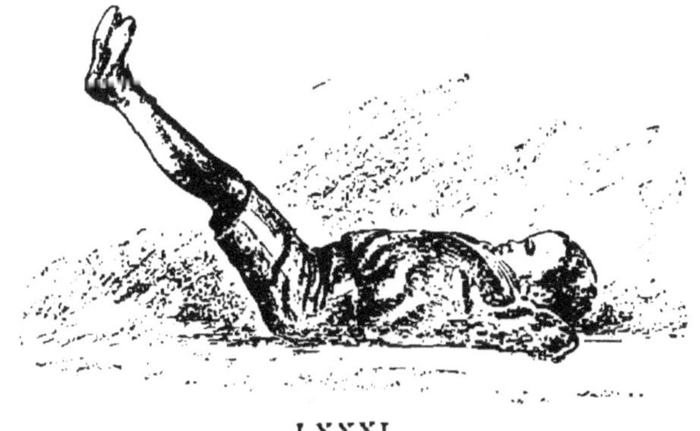

LXXXI.

Lateral Trunk Movement.—Chest-lying; feet fixed; neck firm; head and shoulders raise; *trunk bend.* (2–7 repetitions.)

The movement is the same as the corresponding one in lesson I., recumbent posture, for children. The neck firm posture makes it a very difficult one, and great care should be used that elbows are held in line of shoulder-blades, and that the face is raised in the plane of the wall.

If good posture cannot be maintained from this arm position, continue the movement from hips firm position for a few weeks longer.

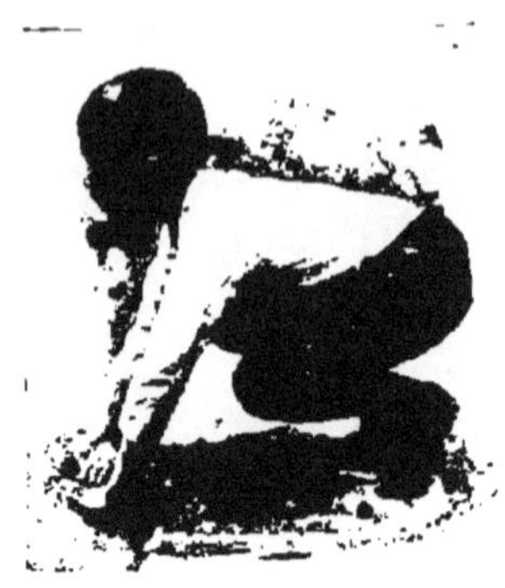
LXXXII.

FOOT MOVEMENT.—As described at beginning. (10 repetitions.)

RESPIRATORY MOVEMENT.—As described at beginning. (10 repetitions.)

A good substitute for the back and abdominal movements is shown in postures LXXXII. and LXXXIII. From the former posture the

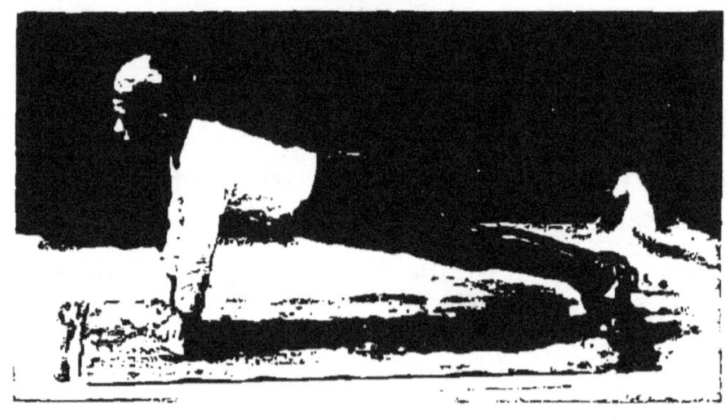
LXXXIII.

child springs to the latter, holding the trunk in suspension, hands and toes only touching the floor. The posture is held a few moments, and the child either springs to former position, or flexes elbows until the simple chest-lying posture is reached. (3–8 repetitions.)

Use care that the trunk does not sag at the waist and that knee muscles are tense. This movement employs well the spinal, chest, and abdominal muscles.

After a few weeks' practice, the movement may be progressed by alternately flexing and extending the elbows (2–5 repetitions from posture LXXXIII.), and after assuming posture LXXXII. for a few moments' rest, repeating the movement.

Further progression includes leg raise, from posture LXXXIII., directing the energy to the extremities of the raised leg. (Repeat 3–5 times with each.)

Later, combine the two; *i. e., spring to posture LXXXIII.; flex elbows;* and from that posture, *raise leg, foot extended.* (3–5 repetitions.)

MEMORANDUM OF PRESCRIPTION II—RECUMBENT POSTURE MOVEMENTS

Children

Respiratory Movement.—To be selected from previous prescriptions.

Chest Raising.—Chest-lying ; feet fixed ; arms upwards bend ; head and shoulders raise ; *arm extension sideways.* (5 repetitions, rest ; 5 repetitions, rest.)

Foot Movement.—Lying ; *foot parting.* (10 repetitions.)

Back Movement.—Chest-lying ; feet fixed ; neck firm ; *head and upper spine raise.* (3–8 repetitions.) Or, *arm pulling in line with trunk.* (2 repetitions, rest ; 2 repetitions, rest ; 2 repetitions, rest ; increase to 5 repetitions.)

Abdominal Movement.—Lying ; neck firm ; head and shoulders raise ; *trunk bend.* (2–7 repetitions each.)

Lateral Trunk Movement.—Chest-lying ; feet fixed ; neck firm ; head and shoulders raise ; *trunk bend.* (2–7 repetitions each.)

Foot Movement.—As mentioned above.

Respiratory Movement.—As mentioned above.

CHAPTER XIX

PRESCRIPTIONS FOR CHILDREN (*Continued*)

"Men are but children of a larger growth."—DRYDEN.

PRESCRIPTION II. — EXERCISE FROM STANDING POSTURE. TO ALTERNATE WITH, OR USE IN PLACE OF, PRESCRIPTION II., RECUMBENT POSTURE FOR CHILDREN.

GUARD carefully against careless chest posture in every movement.

RESPIRATORY MOVEMENT.—*Arms sideways raise, inhaling.* (10 repetitions.) Described in prescription I.

FOOT MOVEMENT.—Neck firm; *foot place forward* (3 repetitions); also *backward* (3 repetitions). Described in lesson II. for adults.

Or, *place outward*, and *backward-outward.* (3 repetitions each.) Described in lesson III. for adults.

In the backward-outward placing, guard against throwing the shoulders back. Use care that the trunk is not twisted nor inclined.

After a few weeks' practice, add *heels raise* to the foot-placings, taking care that the trunk is poised equally on both feet, and neither inclined nor twisted.

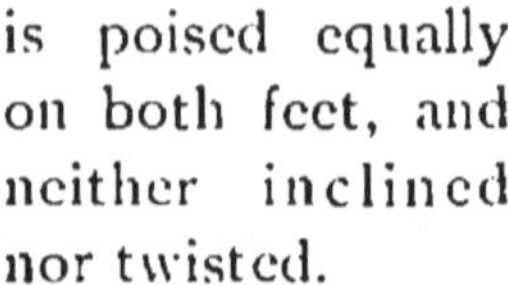

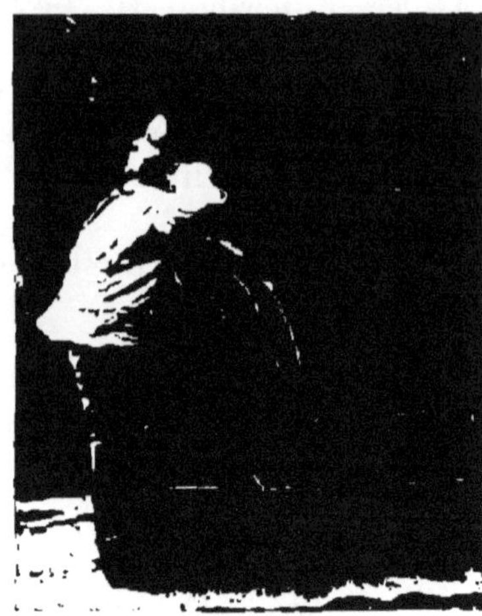

LXXXIV.—CHEST MOVEMENT.

HEAD MOVEMENT.—*Head twist.* (5 repetitions.) Described in lesson I., adults.

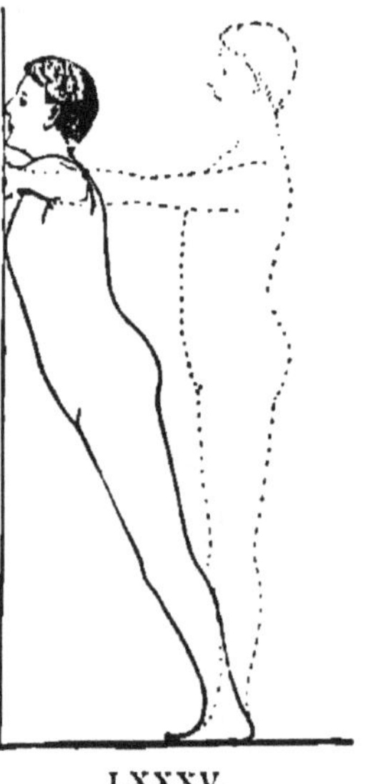

LXXXV.

CHEST MOVEMENT.—Stride-kneeling against shoulder-pressure; neck firm; *head and upper spine backward bend.* (5–8 repetitions.) (Posture LXXXIV.)

Or, standing arm's length from the wall, hands against the wall; *arms bend slowly*, bringing chin and chest in near touch to the wall, bending only from ankles. (5–12 repetitions.)

SHOULDER-BLADE MOVEMENT. — Arms stretch sideways; and from that position, *arm circling*. (10–15 repetitions.) Described in lesson II., adults.

Use care that the head does not push forward during practice of movement.

Vary this with *alternate arm stretch upward and sideways; i. e.*, arms upward bend; *left arm upward, right arm sideways stretch; arms bend* and *stretch* in alternate order; *i. e.*, left arm sideways, right arm upward. (10 repetitions.) Described in prescription II., adults, posture XLIX.

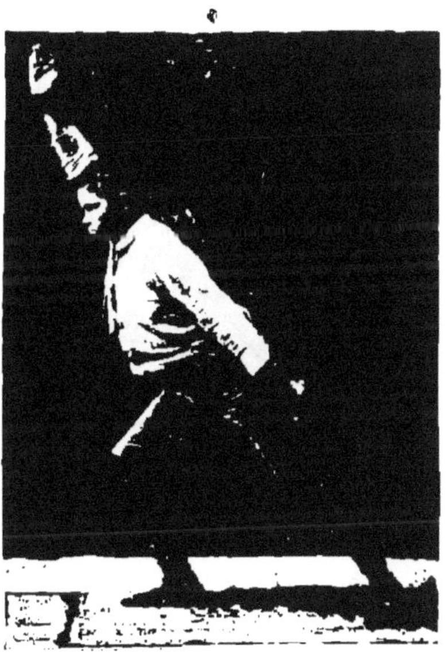

LXXXVI.

Or, arms upward bend; *right arm upward, left arm backward stretch*, and *right forward fall-out.* Described in prescription III., adults. Take care that good position of head and chest is maintained, and that trunk does not twist. (8–15 repetitions.)

BÁLANCE MOVEMENT. — Arms sideways raise; *leg sideways raise.* (3–5 repetitions.) Described in prescription III., posture LVII.

Or, neck firm; *knee upward bend;* hold posture; *backward stretch;* hold posture; *upward bend;* hold posture; *downward* place. (5 repetitions.) Described in prescription II., adults. Take care that trunk does not incline forward. This combines posture XLIII., chapter XII., and posture L., chapter XIII.

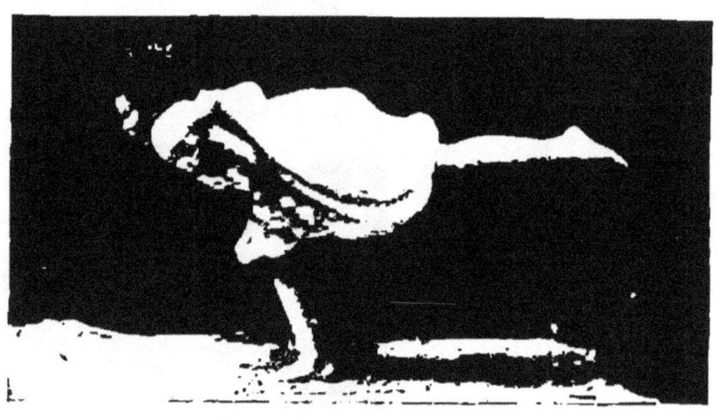

LXXXVII.

In subsequent practice, incline the trunk forward in line with the extended leg, bringing trunk and leg to horizontal position, bending the supporting knee to angle of ninety degrees. Take care that extended foot is well forced (posture LXXXVII.). Hold a few moments, and gradually resume former position. (3-5 repetitions for each leg.)

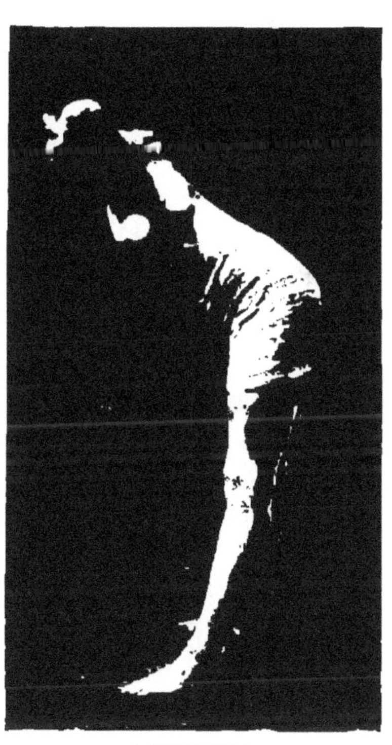

LXXXVIII.

The progression in this movement is in arm posture. Hips firm; arms raised in plane of shoulders; neck firm; arms stretched in line with trunk.

BACK MOVEMENT.--Stride-standing; neck firm; *trunk forward bend*. (5-12 repetitions.) Aim to reach angle of ninety degrees (trunk and legs), maintaining good position of shoulder-blades and chest.

Or, arms upward stretch; *trunk forward-downward bend.* (2-5 repetitions.) Described in prescription III., adults.

ABDOMINAL MOVEMENT. — Lying; neck firm; *legs raise* simultaneously; *knees bend; stretch; legs downward sink.* (3–5 repetitions.) Do not attempt this until good practice on the more simple movement has continued many weeks. The movement is more satisfactorily executed if the elbows are held down firmly by attendant.

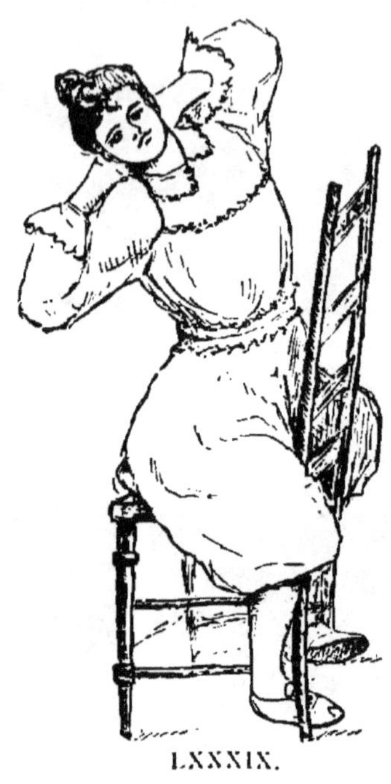
LXXXIX.

LATERAL TRUNK MOVEMENT. — Stride-kneeling or stride-sitting; neck firm; trunk twist; and from that posture *bend.* (5–8 repetitions.) Described in prescription II., adults.

Be careful that the head does not push forward, that elbows are held in line, and that the bend movement is directly under the arm-pit.

JUMP MOVEMENT.—With one, two, or three start-steps, *jump forward.* (5–8 repetitions.)

Or, *outward* or *sideways.* Also *jump down from a stair*, using care to land correctly, and to attain perfect repose of posture before normal position is assumed. Further progression in the jump movement may be attained by combining the start-steps and the landing at an angle of ninety or one hundred and eighty degrees from former plane of the body; also by calculating distance for different number of start-steps. Alternate the start from one foot to the other.

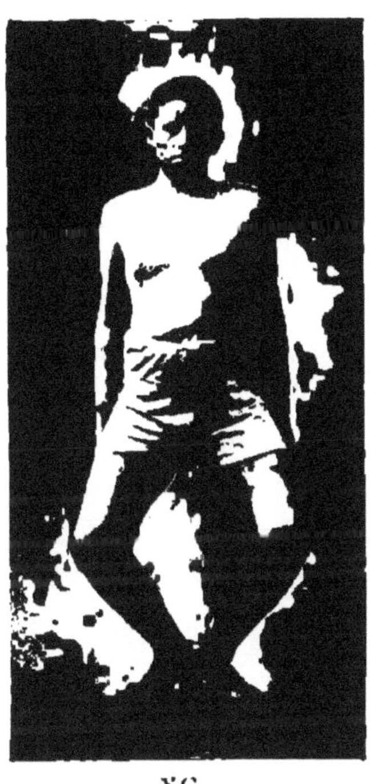

XC.

In place of this, a short run is often recommended, running on toes, and holding head and chest erect.

SLOW LEG MOVEMENT.—Neck firm; *heels raise.* (10 repetitions.)

RESPIRATORY MOVEMENT.—*Arms forward-*

upward raise, inhaling; sideways, hands turn at shoulder height, downward sink, exhaling. (10 repetitions.) Guard against tendency to push the head forward on the upward raise of the arms; upward position of the arms must be in line with the head, trunk, and legs; hands shoulder width apart, and palms directly toward each other. Described in prescription II., adults.

A valuable substitute for the back and abdominal movement is the movement described at the close of prescription II., recumbent posture movements for children. It employs all the muscles on the front, back, and sides of the trunk.

MEMORANDUM OF PRESCRIPTION II—STANDING POSTURE

CHILDREN

RESPIRATORY MOVEMENT.—*Arms sideways raise, inhaling.* (10 repetitions.)

FOOT MOVEMENT. — Neck firm ; *foot place forward* (5 repetitions) ; also *backward* (5 repetitions). Alternate with *outward* and *backward-outward placings.* (5 repetitions each.)

Later, add *heels raise.*

CHEST MOVEMENT. — Stride-kneeling against shoulder-pressure ; neck firm ; *head and upper spine backward bend.* (8–12 repetitions.)

SHOULDER-BLADE MOVEMENT.—*Arm circling.* (12 repetitions.)

Or, *alternate arm stretchings upward and sideways.* (10 repetitions.)

Or, *alternate arm stretchings* and *fall-outs.*

BALANCE MOVEMENT.—Arms raised sideways ; *leg sideways raise.* (3–5 repetitions.)

Or, neck firm ; *knee, upward bend ;* hold ; *backward stretch ;* hold ; *upward bend ;* hold ; *downward place.* (5 repetitions each.)

Approach horizontal poise of trunk and extended leg.

BACK MOVEMENT.—Stride-standing ; neck firm ; *forward bend.* (5–12 repetitions.)

Or, arms stretched upward ; *trunk forward-downward bend.* (2–5 repetitions.)

ABDOMINAL MOVEMENT.—Lying; neck firm; *legs raise; knees bend; stretch: downward sink.* (3–5 repetitions.)

LATERAL TRUNK MOVEMENT.—Stride-kneeling or sitting; neck firm; trunk twist; from that posture, *bend to same side.* (5–8 repetitions.)

JUMP MOVEMENT.—With one, two, or three start-steps, *jump*, landing in toe-knee-bend position. (5–8 repetitions.)

Or, *run.*

SLOW LEG MOVEMENT.—Neck firm; *heels raise.* (10 repetitions.)

RESPIRATORY MOVEMENT.—*Arms forward-upward raise, inhaling: sideways-downward sink, exhaling.* (10 repetitions.)

CHAPTER XX

PASSIVE TREATMENT FOR DELICATE CHILDREN, AND SHORT PRESCRIPTION OF VIGOROUS EXERCISE

"Nature knows no pause in progress and development, and attaches her curse on all inaction."—GOETHE.

WE should be especially careful not to overtax the strength of thin-blooded, nervous children, hence massage and simple passive movements are best for them. Mal-nutrition is generally the cause of their delicate health, and the aim in the manipulations is to improve the functions of the circulatory, respiratory, and digestive organs, without taxing strength, and, by increasing the capillary circulation, to build up the lacking tissues.

Physicians sometimes order olive oil and sometimes cod liver oil (adding, in some cases, a few drops of oleate of quinine), to be used with massage for emaciated children. The oil prevents chafing of the skin from the massage, and renders the treatment more agreeable to a nervous child ; it also nourishes the system somewhat, by absorption through the pores of the skin.

The massage should be very thorough when oil is used; it must be continued longer than without it, as the oil must be well worked into the pores of the skin, and well dried by thorough manipulations so that the pores are not obstructed by it. The skin feels soft and dry after the treatment thus given is completed.

The child should then have some nourishing drink, and absolute rest should follow.

Study well the manipulations described in the chapter on Massage. If there is any especial weakness of throat, chest, or stomach, stimulate the circulation there by a dash of cold water, and then apply the necessary hand manipulations. The cold water application may be omitted or adopted at discretion. (See chapter on Bathing.)

The treatment is as follows:

1. Apply massage first to the extremities; the twist for the legs, and rotation for the feet and joints. Upward stroking to empty the veins follows.

2. The same work is next given for the arms and hands.

3. Apply massage next for the back and sides. This should be very thorough, as stimulation of spinal nerves and of the circulation in spinal and intercostal muscles exerts great influence in the improvement of health.

4. Manipulations for front of the body follow, and are as follows: gentle rotation for chest; stomach rotation; light percussion of liver; rotation for small intestine; stroking of colon.

5. Repeat treatment for legs and arms.

6. Respiratory movement follows. This may be a gentle arm pulling overhead, making the movement in about the rhythm of slow breathing. (10 repetitions.)

Or, grasp patient's shoulders and raise the chest during the inhalation, and allow it to sink to former position during the exhalation.

This is also a good prescription for invalids.

SHORT PRESCRIPTION OF VIGOROUS EXERCISE FOR BED-TIME PRACTICE

To be used in Place of Preceding Ones when Less Time is Advisable

Children

Back and Shoulder-blade Movement.—Chest-lying; feet fixed; head and shoulders raise; *arm extension sideways.* (8 repetitions.)

Or, same posture, *arm pulling in line with trunk.* (5–8 repetitions.) (See Back Movement, chapters XVI. and XVIII.) Be careful that the head is raised, and the face held in plane of the wall, during the execution of the movement. Harm rather than advantage will result from carelessness in small details.

Abdominal Movement.—Lying; neck firm; *legs raise.* (3–8 repetitions.) (See Abdominal Movement, chapter XVIII.)

Lateral Trunk Movement.—Chest-lying; feet fixed; hips firm; head and shoulders raise; *bend to side.* (3–8 repetitions each.) (See Side Movement, chapter XVI.) Followed by cross-wise rubbing of the back, downward stroking, and heavy stroking downward, close against the spine. (See chapter on Massage.)

Later, the same movement from neck-firm posture. (See chapter XVIII.)

Respiratory Movement.—Lying; *arm pulling in line*

with trunk. (10 repetitions.) Attendant will grasp child's hands and slowly and steadily draw them overhead, requesting the child to "breathe in." During the exhalation the arms are returned to bend posture. (See chapter XVI., beginning movement.)

FOOT MOVEMENT.—Neck firm; *bend and stretch ankles.* (10 repetitions.) (See posture LXIII., chapter XV.)

NOTE.—Dr. Gustaf Zander of Stockholm has invented and perfected a system of machines which execute for the individual all the Swedish movements, both active and passive. There are about one hundred of these different machines, based on a carefully estimated plan of leverage and resistance, and so arranged on a scale of progression that individual strength may be accurately used. We boast a fully equipped Zander Institute in New York, at Nos. 9, 11, and 13 East Fifty-ninth Street.

CHAPTER XXI

SELF-DIAGNOSIS

"Know thyself."

THE lessons outlined in the preceding chapters are arranged on a careful scale of progression. The repetitions of the movements are arranged in each lesson in proper proportion for symmetrical development, but are not specific for individual conditions. Advice is given in each prescription, regarding the adaptation of the work to individual conditions, and great advantage is sure to result from it, in the restoration of disused muscles to functional activity, and also, in many cases, in improvement of organic health. Something more, however, is necessary for many women who, through lack of self-knowledge, have contracted ailments more or less severe and threatening.

Disease means derangement of tissues (see quotation from Dr. Lee, chapter VIII.), and may be either chronic or acute. It is chronic when tissues undergo a slow change in their properties, such as in gout, articular rheumatism, and we may also include obesity. Acute disease, as now understood, is caused by the introduction of some poison germ. It is usually characterized by suffering and symptoms that mark certain stages, and terminate after running a certain course (the length of which is usually determined by the patient's conditions), in recovery, death, or invalidism.

Disease needs the physician's attention; but in the incipient stage of many of the common ills, the application of self-massage and the practice of the right plan of movements, with sufficient intervals of rest, simplified diet, and fresh air in abundance, will tend greatly toward allaying the ailment, if not entirely removing it.

Except in cases of organic heart trouble or pelvic weakness, the plan of exercises outlined in this work can be safely followed; provided, of course, the directions be accurately carried out.

The health seeker should adapt the exercises from diagnostic memoranda, both from self-study and with the physician's aid, if heart or pelvic weakness is present.

THESE MEMORANDA COVER:

Age.—In classing conditions as affected by years the following is a good scale, viz.:

1. Infants to one or two years of age.
2. Children to eleven or twelve years.
3. The adolescent period, between the ages of eleven or twelve, and twenty-three or twenty-five.
4. From that age until about forty years of age.
5. Between the ages of forty and fifty.
6. From fifty on.

Anything more specific than this in age is unnecessary, as conditions rather than years influence physique.

Weight and *height* for growing children, in proportion to their age.

Weight and *height* of adults in case of excess or lack of proportionate weight.

Chest expansion.—Pass the tape around the chest under the arms, and, holding it fairly tight, note the difference between the chest contracted by exhalation, and expanded by inhalation. Flexible chest walls admit of three to five inches expansion. The same test should be made around the lower chest, about the ninth rib.

The shoulder girth and *hips girth* should be about equal to each other, and the *waist girth* should be about ten inches less. * Fortunately we have no standard of proportions as an eye-mark, hence no one will suffer by comparison. Every well-developed symmetrical figure is the American Venus.

Chest.—Note whether it is high and well-developed, or flat, or hollow and bony.

Shoulders should be even, and the shoulder-blades snug against the back, not protruding like "wings."

Spine.—Study the chapter on Spine for tests of simple lateral curvature. Study also the normal curves of the spine, and note whether or not these have become exaggerated, allowing shoulders to round, as the saying goes. If the hips are too far forward, the spine will be too nearly straight from the waist down, and the abdomen will protrude.

Development.—Note if the muscles are well proportioned. If there is an excess of adipose, note where it lies.

Circulation.—Note whether or not it is good in the extremities; also if sensitiveness to cold is experienced.

* *Sleep.*—Note if sleep is easily induced, and

is refreshing; or if dreams or restlessness cause fatigue on awakening.

Appetite.—The appetite should be even, and should crave wholesome foods. (See chapter on Digestion.)

Colds.—Note if there is susceptibility to colds, and whether in the head, throat, or chest.

Headache.—Note the nature, whether congestive, neuralgic, from disordered digestion, or weak eyes, and aim to understand the cause. Indigestion, over-mental strain, lack of fresh air and of exercise, or pelvic weakness is liable to lie at the foundation.

Nervousness may take the form of depression, irritability, or collapse. The same causes producing headaches are often responsible for this defect.

Indigestion.—Note whether it is acidity, distension, or lack of assimilation; and whether the cause lies in too little fresh air and exercise, or in imprudence in bathing, eating, or dressing.

Constipation.—The causes may be those mentioned with indigestion, or there may be weak pelvic conditions. (See chapter on Massage; also note advice on hemorrhoids.)

Backache.—Note the location of suffering; it

may be due to many causes. Imprudent dressing (heavy skirts, stiff waist clothing, or high heels), careless posture, over-taxed nerves, congestive headaches, or pelvic weakness are among the most common causes.

Rheumatism.—Note the nature, whether inflammatory or articular. The cause is probably too little exercise of the right kind, and imprudent dietary and dress.

Neuralgia.—Note the location; too little repose, mal-nutrition, or imprudent dressing and bathing is doubtless the cause.

Catarrh.—That of the throat and nose is prevalent in our northern climate. (See chapter on Massage.) Stomach and intestinal catarrh are also common ills, and may be largely relieved by self-knowledge and care.

Ears.—Obstructions and noises in ears are often due to throat catarrh.

Eyes.—Test eyes, and note if any irregularity of vision exists. A simple test is to cover each eye in turn, and see if as accurate reading can be done with the one as with the other. Irregular vision is often the cause of headache, nervous fatigue, etc.

Throat.—Note if there is tendency to irritation, catarrh, tonsilitis, etc.

Lungs.—Note any tendency to weakness, and the cause of such. Weak lungs are liable to be injured by too vigorous respiratory movements.

Pelvic organs.—Any weak conditions of these organs should command attention of the specialist, in the early stages. It is impossible to judge conditions accurately from symptoms. Retroversion is often mistaken for anteversion; and weak tendencies of those tissues are apt to involve complications which even the specialist must watch for and endeavor to prevent. Displacement is often the fate of tired girls and women. If they are educated in self-knowledge, there will be no mistaken ideas of delicacy in seeking necessary advice. Backaches, headaches, dragged looks, and nervous suffering are sure to attend this irregularity of health. Womanhood should not be attended by physical pain. Let every girl be taught this, and taught to understand nature's requirements.

Liver.—An inactive liver is usually evident in complexion and temper. The well-exercised individual need never be conscious of one.

Bladder and *kidneys.*—Note if there are abnormal conditions of these organs. The physician's advice had best be sought.

Heart action.—Irregularity of action may be due to unhygienic habits of dress and diet. It is especially important to consult good medical authority in regard to this, as with the pelvic organs.

Heredity.—This study involves the family record for at least four generations. Understanding the tendencies to disease, one can so shape the influences that surround every-day life as to avoid their development, and can induce length of useful years, often exceeding those of the individual who boasts longevity as his heritage.

Make memorandum from self-diagnosis, as explained, and base the arrangement of lessons and prescriptions upon it, not only in regard to posture, but to localized work, massage, and repetitions of the movements.

Each Swedish lesson and prescription involves the general beginning work, as for the members; localized work, as for trunk muscles; and generalized work in closing.

In the localized work, begin each movement mildly, and add energy gradually with each repetition until near the completion, when a gradual lightening is necessary. By this means the circulation is encouraged, but not forced, in weak tissues.

Posture during practice also affects the therapeutic influence of the movements, and should be as carefully studied as the movements themselves. If fatigued from standing, walking, or bicycling, or in case of weak abdominal organs, the recumbent postures are preferable, for obvious reasons. Half-lying is better than lying, in case of a tendency to excess of blood in the head. Hook-lying or half-lying is preferable for early practice, in case of weak abdominal walls, as lying places them on too continuous a stretch. Either of these three postures should be assumed in anteversion; and chest-lying in cases of retroversion. Prolapsed conditions are improved by all the recumbent postures, but of course either the knee-chest, or lying, hips raised, is best.

In all cases of defective physique it is necessary to understand the cause before applying any specific remedies. Chronic constipàtion, when occasioned by inactivity of the digestive apparatus, should have the work localized to the weakened tissues. Stomach rotation and liver percussion are always necessary, and manipulation of the colon is also essential. Temporary relief from the enema (see chapter on Home Nursing) may be of great advantage; and fresh air, fruit diet, and exercise are also needed, else the manipulations are of but little permanent advantage.

Walking is not considered good exercise when the intestine is distended with fæces.

For reduction of adipose, see chapter on Regulation of Flesh.

Many persons weary themselves and their friends by continually dwelling on their maladies, a habit which is of itself a mental disease, and one requiring treatment.

This advice on self-study will not tend to create or encourage morbid fancies of disease. It will rather aid women in understanding themselves better, and show how to prevent slight ills, and the need of good, prompt medical aid when disease is present. It is to help establish perfect health through the understanding, to prevent the small inroads made upon it in daily life, and to aid in the recognition of functional retardation as distinguished from organic disease.

Many consider that "perfect health" means the ability to drag about the daily routine of life and indifferently perform the noble duties that are necessarily allotted to them. They acknowledge the constant presence of headaches, indigestion, etc., but apologize for them as the "fate of humanity." If they but knew that consciousness of the existence of any organ shows impaired health in it, and that the possibility of prevention lies with themselves, much of their needless bodily suffering would be spared.

We must not allow ourselves to become slaves to disease, but, remembering the words of La Rochefoucauld—"Preserving the health by too strict a regimen is a wearisome malady"—should endeavor to strike a happy medium by the use of our intelligence.

CHAPTER XXII

MASSAGE

"We ought to be thankful to Nature for having made these things which are necessary, easy to be discovered."—EPICURUS.

THE art of massage is as old as humanity itself; and although for centuries it shared the fate of all sciences, and lay comparatively dormant, research shows that at no time has it fallen into complete disuse. There are traces of its practice found in the records and traditions of all nations, civilized and savage, through the different ages of history.

Within the last four or five hundred years, a revival of this almost lost art has set in. The works of Descartes, of Newton, of the famous Bacon, and of Borelli placed massage on a foundation of good authority; and, later on, in the eighteenth century, the celebrated Hoffman, in his "Dissertations Physico-Medicæ," and Francis Fuller's "Medicina Gymnastico," which Kleen characterizes as "an echo from Hoffman," gave a much needed impetus to the movement. Tissot of France was another valuable exponent.

In the estimation of many, the art lies alone in the manipulation. No greater error than this can exist, and serious injuries to health are liable to result when the invalid (or semi-invalid, I will say) is subjected to treatment so superficially grounded. The *masseuse* needs, as foundation for the study of this art, a physician's preparation in anatomy and physiology, and also a good course of instruction in therapeutics. She will then be able not only to comprehend the theory of the influence manipulations have on disease, but to understand the location of blood-vessels and nerve-trunks, and to conduct with intelligence the treatment with reference to such influence. She will also be able to adapt it to organic conditions for the healthy as well as for those physically defective, an essential every patient should demand. Too much care cannot be given to the assimilation of a prescription of massage to meet the complications of defects common to most Americans. It were a boon to humanity were more physicians working on these lines, and fewer in *materia medica*; and it will be a still more tangible boon to humanity when all our physicians recognize, as a few do now, that only skilled labor should be employed in this art. Even with intelligent, well-educated, scrupulous manipulators, the work should go hand-in-hand with the physician's. The manipulator must be able to detect signs of fatigue, and adjust the work and rest periods accordingly, and must be able to distinguish real improvement from nerve exhilaration. She should also report, from time to time, the patient's condition to the physician.

Another common mistake regarding massage is that the technique can be learned from books. Theory can, of course, be ably placed on paper; but even that, to be of advantage, should be interpreted to the student by an experienced instructor. Consider what place it is holding in its influence on human suffering, and you will see that the medical student can as well dispense with instructions in the course of his preparation as the *masseuse* in hers.

Laying theory aside, technique of massage cannot possibly be obtained, except, as in piano work, through practical instructions, and in classes sufficiently small for each member to receive practical work upon the person. The touch can then be imitated, and skill attained through practice. The student needs months of practice in order to attain skill, and the instructor should frequently review the work by personal touch in order to correct errors in technique. Conscientious criticism should be scrupulously given before the student receives her diploma and is sent out on her mission of benefiting humanity. Until skilled labor is demanded by the physicians and people, the ignorant and the superficially prepared will continue to dupe humanity by pretending to pursue the noble art.

Let them call their work rubbing, not massage.

A *masseuse* should always possess a calm temperament. The work is not of advantage if given by irritable, restless manipulators, especially for nervous Americans.

The work should never be overdone, and the patient should always feel comfortable after treatment. If discomfort follows, a person well versed in the science should be consulted before treatment—even the simple work described here—is continued.

In this chapter I shall, of course, attempt no description of scientific manipulations, but have substituted for such, simpler methods, adapted for home use, and which, if properly applied, will go far toward checking ills in their incipiency, and toward preventing the recurrence of common ills. Although they should accompany movements, as suggested in the prescriptions of exercise, much good follows their independent use.

Breathing movements should follow the manipulations, and the blood should be directed to the extremities after the treatment for the head and trunk is completed. Rest should follow, and it must be remembered that rest does not mean merely assuming recumbent posture. It means cessation from all thought. Rest! Let it be a sacred text for American women.

A careful perusal of the chapters on Circulation, Respiration, and Digestion is necessary in order to interpret the theory suggested in this one.

The aim in massage is to improve the capillary and venous circulation and to stimulate the nerves. For joints and irregular-shaped muscles a rotary movement is employed. Place the hand, or the palmar surfaces of finger-ends, in touch upon the part needing massage, and by a rotary motion move the skin on the muscle, not occasioning friction of skin. The movement is not necessarily rapid. The amateur should give no manipulation for sensitive joints, unless the treatment is sanctioned by a physician.

The capillary circulation in the long muscles is stimulated by rubbing them crosswise their length, both hands being used in close touch, but moving in opposite directions. The movement is preferably slow, but must be firm and steady.

After stimulating the capillaries, the veins should be emptied; this is done by stroking heavily on the large veins toward the heart. (See illustrations XCI., XCII., and XCIII.) The veins thus emptied fill from the lesser ones, and these from lesser branches, and so on in the grade of the subdivisions, until the smallest are reached; and these fill from the capillaries, which receive in place of the venous blood a fresh supply of arterial blood. Veins are provided with valves that prevent their filling, except in the one direction.

The rubber rollers are helpful in self-massage, and they also help the attendant greatly in giving treatment for back and limbs.

I will explain the applied work.

Congestive Headaches.—The movement is made with the palmar surfaces of the fingers, and is necessarily vigorous. Begin on top of the head, and continue the treatment backward and downward to base of the brain; continue also from the temples backward and downward. Much and heavy rotation at base of brain should follow; also crosswise rubbing on the back of the neck, and stroking from the head down back of the ears to the shoulders, for the purpose of emptying the veins. A foot movement (see prescriptions of exercise) or arm massage should follow, to draw the blood to the extremities and thus relieve pressure in the head. It is best in severe cases to have passive foot movement and arm massage precede, as well as follow, the head treatment.

The tendency to congestive headaches may be greatly lessened by dashes of very cold water at back of neck and down the spine before the morning bath.

Neuralgic Headaches.— These require gentler massage than that prescribed for congestive headaches. Complete rest is often all that is necessary. Headaches arising from malnutrition are relieved by the stomach treatment. Remember, in every ailment, treatment must

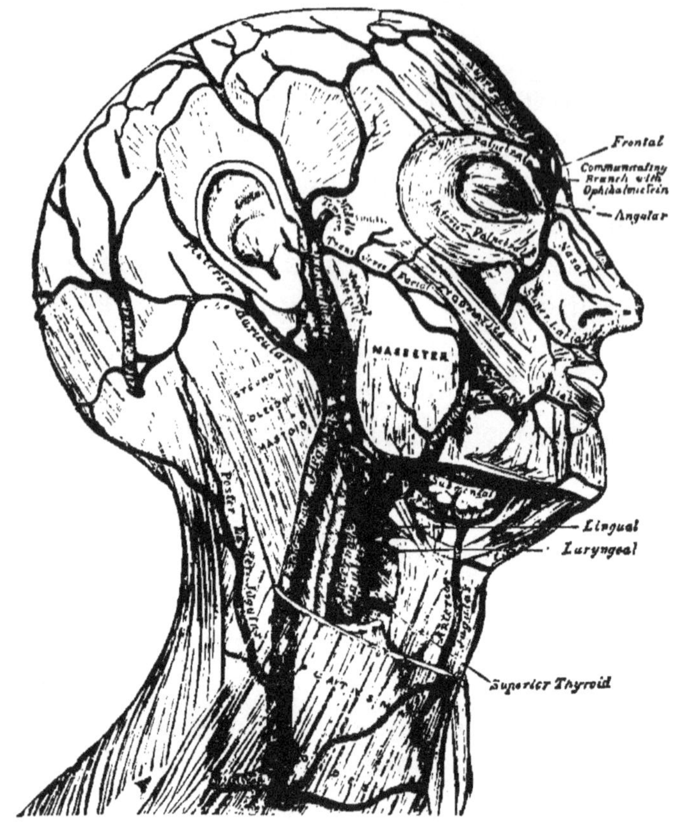

XCI. Showing Large Veins of the Head.

be intelligently conducted from a knowledge of the cause.

Nasal Catarrh.—The manipulation employed for this consists in placing a finger (the second is most convenient) of each hand on either side of the nose at the union of the bone and cartilage, making rapid rotation, having first moistened the lining of the nose with vaseline, or a cold cream containing only pure ingredients.

It is also of great benefit to take nasal douches night and morning; more frequently if desired. Warm water softened with a little glycerine (a half teaspoonful to a cup of water) is a universally safe and satisfactory bath to use, and may be snuffed up, if the patient prefers it to using a tube.

The treatment is also valuable in case of colds in the head or throat.

Weak Throats.—For strengthening the tissues of the throat we employ first a crosswise rubbing, placing the hands (thumbs backward) on the throat, and allowing them to pass each other in reciprocal movement. Do not lift the hands from the throat between the strokings. Moisten the skin with vaseline, if necessary, to prevent irritation. This movement can be done to excellent advantage by the patient, but the service of an attendant gives better results. When an attendant gives the treatment, the patient reclines, and the attendant stands back of the chair or at the head of the couch, thereby making both posture and movement convenient to each. Follow the stroking by rotation at the base of the neck. The entire right hand is employed in this manipulation. Place the base of the forefinger in the clavicular notch, and move the skin on the tissues underneath, making first a slow circle and increasing in rapidity until it approaches a vibration. It will at first occasion coughing, but this inconvenience will be but temporary. It should be repeated at frequent intervals in case of colds. When a tickling in the throat is experienced, let the patient allay it by this treatment and by sips of cold water, rather than by the harmful habit of coughing and of "scraping" the throat, and permanent good will surely result.

Thin necks are best permanently improved by the exercises, although gentle massage is a valuable agent.

LUNG TISSUE is also benefited by the rotary movement. It should begin at the bifurcation of the bronchial tubes (third rib), and extend in the direction of the main tubes (see cut VIII., chapter V.), taking care that good breathing is maintained meanwhile. Light percussion may also be used to good advantage for the lungs, but the pernicious custom, followed by some, of filling the lungs with air, and percussing while holding the breath, cannot be too strongly denounced. Such a proceeding is not only liable to weaken the tissues and destroy somewhat the contractility of the lung cells, but it also prevents reoxygenation of the blood; and meanwhile the greater demand for oxygen is being created through the stimulation caused by the percussion.

Percussion for the lungs should be light, and should be given with fingers only. It should begin at the bifurcation of the bronchial tubes, and extend, during the inhalation, along the main branches; returning, on the exhalation, to the same point of the chest from which the treatment begins. Light percussion on the sides should follow. If the treatment is given by an attendant, percussion for the upper back had best be added, but it should be accompanied by full breathing.

BACK MUSCLES.—Treatment for the back

can only be done by an attendant, or by the patient in using the roller referred to. The patient should assume a comfortable posture, either chest-lying or prone-sitting. The chest-lying is preferable. The work may be done outside of light clothing if desired, but it is not as beneficial as when next to the skin. In all massage where use of the entire hand is involved, see that the entire surface of the hand remains in touch with the patient, and that equal continuous pressure is given by every part of the hand. If the patient detects lack of confidence in the touch of the *masseuse*, she will derive but little advantage from her work. Such slip-shod work often causes nervousness.

In treatment for the back, the attendant will place her hands side by side and in touch, and will stroke the muscles crosswise, the hands passing each other in reciprocal movement, beginning at the neck and continuing downward. The movement, although not severe, is necessarily heavy, in order to benefit the deep layers of muscles. Follow this by longitudinal stroking downward, and stimulate the spinal nerves by making heavy, deep pressure on each side of the spine and close against it with the side of the thumbs.

In case of especially weak muscles at the waist, frequent crosswise rubbing there will prove very helpful. This can be done by the patient herself. From a prone-standing or prone-sitting posture she can easily reach her back at the waist. This rubbing is restful, even if given outside of the clothing. A dash of cold water on these muscles before the morning bath will help in stimulating the circulation there.

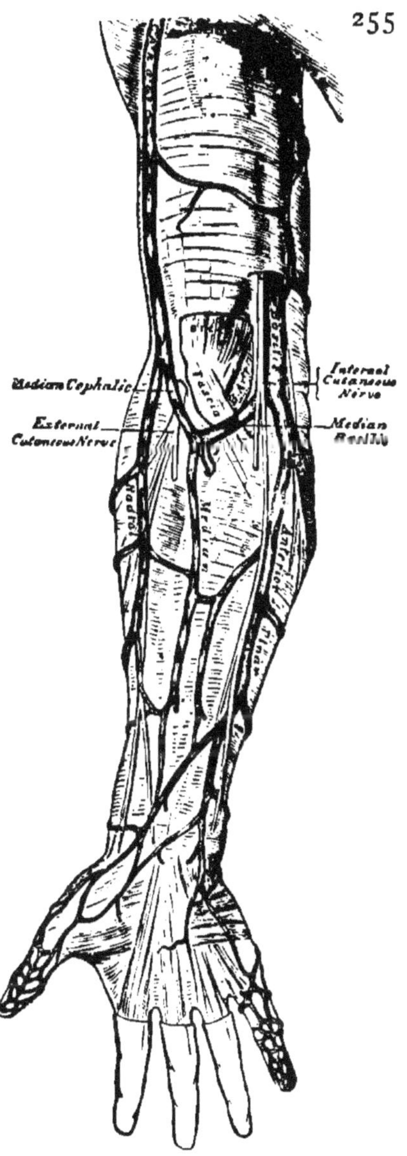

XCII.—Showing Large Veins of the Arm.

ARM MUSCLES.—For improving circulation in these, a crosswise rubbing

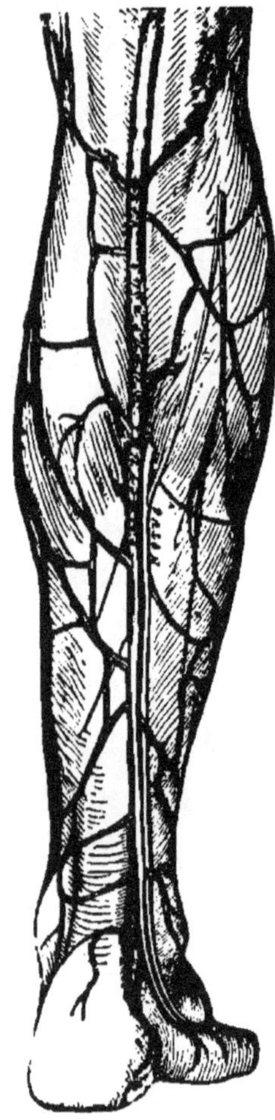

XCIII.
Showing Large Veins of the Leg.

is desirable. This is also done by an attendant; she will grasp with both hands, thumbs towards each other, the patient's arm at the shoulder, and twist the arm muscles by allowing her hands to pass each other in reciprocal movement; continue the movement from shoulder to hand. (5–8 repetitions.) It may be necessary to accompany this by rotation of finger and hand muscles. Stroke heavily to shoulder, making pressure on flexor side of arm, to empty the veins and assist the venous circulation. (5–8 repetitions.)

Leg Muscles are treated similarly, though for the adult the treatment described for the back will be necessary for the thigh; the twist may be used for the legs. Apply treatment first to the front of the legs;

then, when patient assumes chest-lying posture, treatment for back of thighs can be given, followed by heavy stroking to empty veins. It is best to disturb the patient as little as possible by frequent change of posture.

FINGER OR TOE JOINTS.—In case of gouty diathesis it is necessary to give daily attention to the lesser joints, even though no accumulation of calcareous deposit is apparent. Hands and feet are not usually hygienically dressed until the need of care is apparent; hence, I will repeat, give daily attention to strengthening the tissues of joints so that they may be able to resist the unhygienic influence of tight gloves and shoes, which custom at present demands. The patient can treat herself quite successfully. Lay the hand to be manipulated on a firm but not hard support, and placing the side of the other hand on the finger joints perform the rotary movement described, stroking finally toward the shoulder.

For toes, raise the foot to a comfortable position, and placing the palm of one hand under base of toes for support, rotate heavily with the side of the other hand; or, better, with the fist. Stroke upward to empty the veins.

ANKLES AND KNEES.—Place palms of hands

on opposite sides of joint, and rotate, not simultaneously, but each hand following the other in quick succession.

These movements can be done by the patient. They are not to be employed in cases of injured or irritated joints, except on recommendation of a physician.

It is especially important that this general massage be given young infants; and if there are poorly conditioned muscles, additional care should be given them. Drawing the blood through weak tissues several times per day by gentle massage will bring wonderful results in normal development. Irregular features, as a short upper lip, can also be improved by moulding and stretching the muscles during the plastic age.

The bath hour is favorable for baby's massage.

INDIGESTION.—Manipulation for indigestion is clear in theory and simple in execution. If the walls of the stomach are lacking in power, or if the circulation is impaired in the tissues, manipulation will help restore these functions.

Place the left hand neck firm (see description in lessons) so that the muscles in the location of the stomach are placed on a stretch.

Place the right hand on the left short ribs, wrist palm resting on "pit of the stomach." Rotate the skin on the muscles, making a wide circle. The most powerful part of the stroke should be towards the left. Gradually increase the rapidity. A vibration is better than a rotation, on account of its stimulating effect on the nerves. In case of acute suffering at the cardiac orifice, apply friction there, rubbing rapidly up and down with the hand until a burning sensation results. This may take the place of the old-time mustard paste; it produces equally quick relief.

The victim of indigestion must of course make rational dietary her study. She will also obtain much benefit by sipping a cup of hot water night and morning and also an hour before meals. If there is a tendency to acidity of the stomach a half teaspoonful of bicarbonate of soda may be profitably added occasionally.

INACTIVE LIVER.—The liver requires much more vigorous treatment than the stomach does. Place both hands on the right lower chest and side; percuss rapidly, beginning with light force, and increasing at discretion, lightening again before the treatment is completed. (See also Enema, chapter on Home Nursing.)

CHRONIC CONSTIPATION.—In average cases of chronic constipation we aim to stimulate the vermicular motion of the colon, and to restore its functions, which have been interrupted perhaps by imprudence in dress or diet, lack of proper kind of exercise, by colds, or possibly by the indiscriminate use of cathartics or of the enema. It is obviously necessary to treat the cause, else we can induce no permanent advantage. If the cause is among those above mentioned, the manipulations here described will prove invaluable; if from weakness of the pelvic organs, they will not only be of no avail, but may prove positively harmful.

For the manipulation, assume either half-lying or hook-lying position at discretion. (See cuts in Prescription of Recumbent Posture Movements).

If treatment is given next the skin, vaseline had best be used to prevent irritation. Place the fingers of one hand on those of the other, to aid in firmness of pressure, and stroke heavily from lower right side of abdomen upwards to short ribs, across to the short ribs on the left side, and downward to the lower left side of the abdomen; not across from the left to the right side, for obvious reasons. (See chart of Digestive Viscera.) Repeat from 10 to 50 strokes, resting between, if fatigue is experienced. Begin with moderate pressure, and increase, at discretion, to a powerful stroke, providing no internal sensitiveness is noticed. Stroke more lightly before ceasing the manipulation. This may be followed by, or substituted for, if desirable, a double rotation, which is made by the fingers of both hands following each other.

The massage rollers are excellent aids in manipulation of the colon.

It is easily seen, by studying a chart of the human body, that no organs in a person of normal conditions lie directly back of the colon, hence no harm can result from this treatment when only average causes are present. The physician should decide regarding the conditions of the patient's pelvic organs.

In case of sensitiveness at the sigmoid flexure, hold the fingers of the left hand there, making the stroke with right hand only.

Rotating the hand on the small intestine is also of advantage in stimulating vermicular motion.

The enema (see chapter on Home Nursing)

is often employed for temporary relief, in connection with the manipulations.

HEMORRHOIDS are relieved by first pressing the protrusions up into place, and then from prone-stride-sitting posture, or, better, knee-chest posture, percuss the sacral spine heavily with the half-open fist. The motion is from the wrist. (The percussion with closed fist makes too heavy a jar.) This stimulation is of much advantage, and can easily be done by the patient. Bleeding piles are sometimes improved by this percussion. Conditions of this nature should always be reported to the physician, and delay is liable to bring serious results.

KIDNEYS require lighter manipulation than that described for hemorrhoids. Assume prone-stride-standing or sitting posture, and with palmar surfaces of fingers percuss lightly at the waist. (See location of kidneys.)

A dash of cold water, or shower or douche on kidneys or liver is also an excellent stimulation.

CHAPTER XXIII

REGULATION OF FLESH

"Aim at perfection in every thing, though in most things it is unattainable. However, they who aim at it, and persevere, will come much nearer to it than those whose laziness and despondency make them give it up as unattainable." —CHESTERFIELD.

THE thin ask how they may gain weight, and the stout desire to lessen their adipose. Excess in either direction is undesirable, but each condition, like any other physical defect, must be treated from the cause. The same root, mal-assimilation, is liable to be responsible for each evil; and this, according to our best authorities, is due more to a lack of harmonious working of the digestive organs than to indiscriminate selection of foods.

We will first consider those burdened with adipose, and then those of abnormal thinness.

We find many persons of light appetite and of rational dietary gaining adipose steadily. There certainly must be some cause other than dietetic inconsistency for such cases. They are, however, not usual. Generally, we find the stout individual craves foods that tend to increase the weight; and we also find unhealthy conditions existing which cause abnormalities of appetite just as surely as diseased nerve centres demand alcoholic drinks for the inebriate. Perfect health brings desire for healthful foods only. This is explained in the chapter on Digestion.

Adipose consists of globules of fat that have not been utilized as body fuel, hence are stored away for future needs. These needs may be warmth, combustion, or food. In certain quantities, adipose is ever present (except in cases of emaciation, when it has been consumed), and renders comely the angles and hollows that would present themselves were the skin shaped to the muscles without it.

When the blood becomes surcharged with these atoms, nature seeks storage for them in unused parts of the body, where the atoms that have formed flakes in the normal anatomy serve as a nucleus for the massive layers that gradually accumulate, and prove barriers to freedom and comfort. Advice from the physician is sought, regarding cause and remedy.

His verdict gives as the cause too little exercise of the correct kind, and too much fuel food. The remedy lies in ascertaining what the correct exercise is, and performing it, and also in lessening the amount of fat-producing food taken into the system. Clothing that restricts good circulation also causes increase of adipose. I refer to the ligature for stocking support and to tight and stiff waist clothing. Full capillary circulation in muscle fibres is prevented by wearing these; the venous current is also retarded, and fatty deposit is, in consequence, lodged in the tissues, which the muscles would be able to resist were they actively exercised, and allowed their freedom.

Some cases are capable of symmetrical reduction, and some can only be improved, or, perhaps, but checked from further increase. Other conditions are obstinate, yielding to no treatment, save, perhaps, heroic dietary or drugs, whereby health is often seriously impaired, and permanent reduction is even then not certain.

I will quote some of the causes that yield least readily to treatment; but even these are capable of general improvement in health, flexibility, and coördination, and, in consequence, may derive ultimate advantage.

1. Imperfect heart action due to organic insufficiency.

2. Functional interruption of heart action caused by fatty degeneration in the tissues of the circulatory apparatus.

3. Heart action impeded, from chest walls being crowded with adipose.

4. Respiratory insufficiency caused by fatty degeneration of tissues, and also by chest being crowded with adipose.

5. Lack of mental control.

This last is really the most difficult barrier we encounter in reduction treatment. Those who over-eat will continue to indulge their appetites (and we have no Keeley cure for such), and the indolent will not practice systematic exercise. In cases, however, where the palate does not rule, and where organic health is favorable, reduction of adipose is, to a certain extent, sure, providing a correct diagnosis is made, and plans are properly adjusted and followed. The work can be accomplished through the circulation only. The blood has deposited the adipose, atom by atom, and no other agent than the blood can remove it. The removal is necessarily a slow process, atom by atom, as was the accumulation, and involves time and patient practice. It brings its reward in more ways than one. Besides rendering the figure more symmetrical, the muscles more flexible, and improving the circulation, organic health and longevity are promoted.

I state truths here, not fallacies. These marvellous tales of successful reduction in a week's time through "dry diet," are untrue. It is, however, possible, by this means and the aid of doses of sulphate of soda, to reduce the girth in that length of time, as the superfluity of vapors and gases in the digestive viscera that was causing much of the distension is of course lessened by this change of regimen; but no reduction of the adipose itself can be effected in so short a period of time, and through these means. Let this be remembered when records of miraculous reduction are heralded.

Adipose, unlike other tissues of the body, is not supplied with capillaries through which destruction and rebuilding rapidly take place. It is reduced by increasing the combustion, thus bringing a demand on the reserve of fuel. We accomplish this increase of combustion by exercise, which also improves the digestive and muscular systems, and the tissues are thus rendered resistive to a further accumulation.

Further aid is given by taking less fat producing material into the body.

The steam or hot bath, followed by the cold shower or sponge (providing the physician decides the advisability of this treatment) is temporarily helpful in some cases. It increases circulatory and respiratory functions through the influence of the peripheral nerves, and increases oxygenation, and consequently carbonic acid elimination. But the conclusion of our ablest authorities, among whom I will name Baruch, Voit, and Ranke, is that the result is largely in favor of ultimate increase, rather than diminution of weight. Winternitz proves this by tests of several thousand cases in his establishment, fifty-six per cent. of whom gained in weight, thirty per cent. lost, and fourteen per cent. showed no change. Such facts go to prove that the thin woman, rather than the stout, should be subjected to hydrotherapy, and that the stout woman's need of the bath is for cleanliness only. The Turkish bath, while it may regulate the distribution of fatty matter, and temporarily reduce the weight, removes it from the body only by increasing combustion. Fat is not sweated out, as some people erroneously fancy. (See chapter on Systematic Baths.)

When adipose is reduced by aid of exercise, the tissues are rendered firm and resistive; the digestive apparatus is improved, so that food matter is properly utilized, and accumulation of fat need not afterward be feared. When it is reduced by diet, massage, and hot baths, the tissues are not strengthened, and are likely to yield to former conditions again. Exercise that directs the energy to unused muscles is the stout individual's reliable medicine. Walking cannot do this, and walking is often too heavy a tax on organic health.

For authority on dietary for the over-stout, I mention Dr. I. Burney Yeo as the broadest in research of dietetic principles. He quotes the best authorities of the world, and presents the impossibilities of giving specific advice except from individual study and analysis, though he gives general principles, of course.

He names excess of food as a leading cause, and emphasizes this remark by saying that about and after middle age the body needs less food than it did in earlier years, and this fact not being understood by the individual, the appetite is satisfied daily as it was in earlier years, when the tissue building was more active; and that the extra quantity of food not being required for the body's use is stored away in form of adipose.

Ebstein's method recommends the use of fat in foods, because it so soon produces a feeling of satiety or satisfaction, and leads to the consumption of less food. It also lessens the desire for fluids. This is an echo of Hippocrates' teachings.

Specialists generally decide in favor of Oertel's system. He claims that his system not only provides for the removal of fat, but prevents its reaccumulation, and at the same time improves circulatory and other functions. He distinguishes two degrees of obesity—the lesser form, in which circulatory organs are unaffected, and vigorous exercise is advisable; and the graver form, in which the heart muscle is weakened, and vigorous bodily exercise, in consequence, must be avoided. His great idea is to effect cure by strengthening the muscles of the heart by a practice of systematic bodily exercise, and by this and a carefully considered dietary to preserve normal composition of the blood. He mentions lean beef, veal, mutton, game, eggs, green vegetables, as spinach, etc., fat and carbo-hydrates in limited quantities, and from four to six ounces of bread daily as a foundation of food selection. He limits the quantity of fluids to from twenty-six to thirty fluid ounces during the twenty-four hours.

This is a brief of the "Oertel cure" that has been adopted with some modifications by Schweninger.

Germain Lee protests against the limitations of beverages, and urges hot dilutant drinks. He shows the advantage of their solvent power as an aid to digestion, and also the direct need in gouty diathesis. He, however, does not allow alcoholic drinks.

Dr. S. Weir Mitchell advocates rest, milk diet, and massage, and adds that a diet of skimmed milk alone will safely effect a reduction of half a pound per day. He guards the patient carefully from depletion of vital health from insufficient nourishment, and adds beef, chicken, or oyster soup, as needs require. Swedish movements also accompany the massage, and in good time are supplanted by active Swedish exercises, accompanied with more satisfying dietary.

Science has grouped food into three great divisions, and I quote here the table showing the proportionate amount of each in daily diet recommended by our three leading authorities:

	Albuminates.	Fats.	Carbo-hydrates.
Banting:	5 oz.	⅓ oz.	2¾ oz.
Ebstein:	3½ "	3 "	1⅝ "
Oertel:	5½–6 "	1–1¼ "	2½–3½ "

Banting's system is considered unfavorable from its rigorous exclusion of fats, which are essential to healthy nutrition.

Yeo deduces, from a thorough acquaintance with the theories of other authorities, the following:

"The albuminates in the form of animal food should be strictly limited. Farinaceous and all starchy foods should be reduced to a minimum. Sugar should be entirely prohibited. A moderate amount of fats, for the reasons given by Ebstein, should be allowed.

"Only a small quantity of fluid should be permitted at meals, but enough should be allowed to aid in the solution and digestion of the food. Hot water or warm aromatic beverages may be taken freely between meals, or at the end of the digestive process, especially in gouty cases, on account of their eliminative action.

"No beer, porter, or sweet wines of any kind to be taken; no spirit, except in very small quantity. It should be generally recognized that the use of alcohol is one of the most common provocatives of obesity. A little hock, still Moselle, or light claret, with some alkaline table water, is all that should be allowed. The beneficial effects of such a diet will be aided by abundant exercise and by the free use of saline purgatives, so that we may insure a complete daily unloading of the intestinal canal.

"It is only necessary to mention a few other details. Of animal foods, all kinds of lean meat may be taken, poultry, game, fish (eels, salmon, and mackerel are best avoided), eggs.

"Meat should not be taken more than once a day, and not more than six ounces of cooked meat at a time.

"Two lightly boiled or poached eggs may be taken at one meal, or a little grilled fish.

"Bread should be toasted in thin slices, and completely, not browned on the surface merely.

"Hard captain's biscuit may also be taken.

"Soups should be avoided, except a few tablespoonfuls of clear soup.

"Milk should be avoided unless skimmed,

and taken as the chief article of diet. All milk and farinaceous puddings and pastry of all kinds are forbidden.

"Fresh vegetables and fruits are permitted.

"It is important to bear in mind that the actual quantity of food permitted must have a due relation to the physical development of the individual, and that what would be adequate in one case might be altogether inadequate in the case of another person of larger physique."

Yeo recommends a half pint of hot water, taken a half hour before each meal and before bed-time, as a valuable aid, especially where there is gouty tendency, and recommends, with dietetic restrictions, physical exercise as the agent for consuming excess of fat deposited in the body. He also adds that careful consideration of each case must be made. A variety of food must be prescribed, so that no organic weakness will develop from robbing the blood of tissue-building material, as is often the case from too rigid dietary.

I give these theories not for the purpose of advocating any particular one, but to show the divergence of opinion by the ablest writers on the subject of reduction of flesh by dietary.

The chief point of similarity seems to be in the great reduction in amount of starchy foods, the reduction in quantity of all foods, and the suppression of alcohol.

No system of dietary will reduce the flesh in all cases, and any system is incomplete without the aid of carefully prescribed exercises.

The Swedish leaders attach no importance to any system of dietary for this purpose, but rely mainly on systematized exercise.

The best permanent results in my own experience have been attained by making little change in the diet, except in reduction of quantity of food, of starchy foods, and of liquids with the food, and using systematized exercises.

Exercise must be carefully assimilated, and the amount of work prescribed for the stout woman must be in accord with her heart action. Nature fashioned her heart for working a less bulky machine, and we must respect Nature's plan. A well-assimilated prescription of exercise will tend greatly to improve the functions of the vital organs, while overwork of any groups of muscles may seriously impair them. The energy must be localized in overburdened muscles, but general exercise must also receive much attention. Respiratory movements should several times appear on the prescription. This aids combustion by introducing more oxygen into the blood, and, consequently, more destruction of tissue takes place. Massage of face and neck must attend the reduction work, to prevent wrinkles and the withered condition of the skin which is apt to attend a less careful plan.

For reduction work I rely on the following formula. Each lesson and prescription from the lesson chapters of this book can be easily adapted to this, in turn, repeating for the movements which appear more than once in the formula the movements given in the lesson from which selections are taken. Care should be taken not to advance too rapidly into vigorous work. The simple movements should first be well practiced.

1. Respiratory Movement.
2. Foot Movement.
3. Head Movement.
4. Chest Movement.
5. Abdominal Movement.
6. Shoulder-blade Movement.
7. Balance or Foot Movement.
8. Respiratory Movement.

9. Lateral Trunk Movement.
10. Back Movement.
11. Abdominal Movement.
12. Lateral Trunk Movement.
13. Foot Movement.
14. Respiratory Movement.

Additional resistance and additional number of repetitions for the localized work will also prove of great aid; but the prescription must always be based on the individual's heart ac-

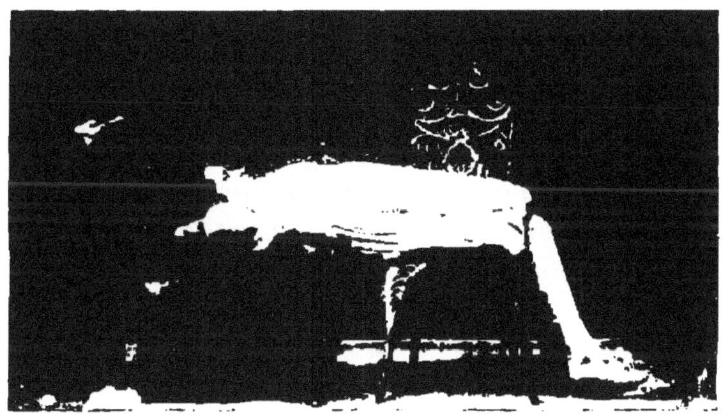

XCIV.

tion, and the posture for practice must be adapted to health of pelvic organs.

The sit-lying posture (XCIV.) adds resistance to abdominal muscles, and may be used to advantage for simple and, later on, more difficult abdominal movements, as *leg raise; leg raise, knee bend* (posture XCV.), and *leg raise* and

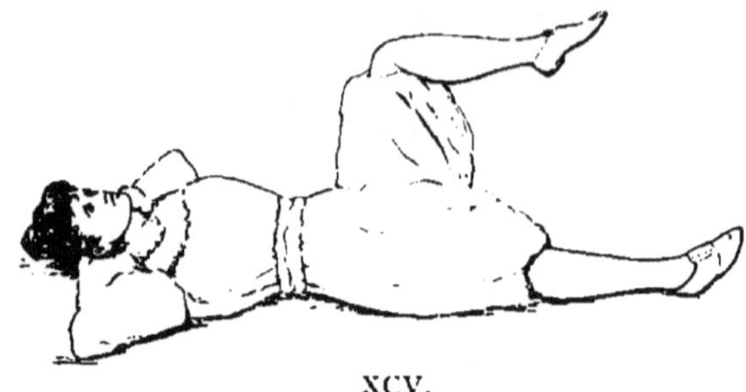

XCV.

circumduct, in order of progression, but should only be approached by weeks of preparatory work.

It is not always possible to effect any perceptible reduction in weight, but it is certain that muscular vigor and the functions of the internal organs are improved, and further accumulation of adipose is checked.

EXTREME LEANNESS.

Extreme leanness is generally considered as undesirable a condition as excess of adipose, and the foundation of good results must rest on elimination of the causes. The thin woman lacks blood; not only in quantity, but in quality. Shall she eat more fuel foods? one asks. Not until the health of her digestive organs has been improved, and nature, in consequence, can utilize such. Shall she exercise less? another will ask. Not less, perhaps, but more wisely. It depends on the cause of her thinness.

I will advise that she read and ponder well the chapter on Fatigue and Rest, for on that hangs the law of her existence. We must rest her, and we must feed her discreetly, in small quantities and frequently. She must also practice systematized exercise, and breathe plenty of fresh air.

Her exercises will probably be passive, and, in any case, they will be milder than those prescribed for her stout sister, though the same general principles are involved. The blood current must be forced through the entire muscular system, and the functions of the body will be thereby increased. Massage, perhaps with oil, will be a valuable remedial agent for her, but it must be of a less vigorous character than that arranged for the stout woman. Turkish baths (providing her heart action permits them) are also valuable aids to tissue growth. I base this on authority of Winternitz.

The thin woman must await patiently the evolution of better conditions. A year must be to her as a single day, which is not generally in accord with her taste. Usually we find her restless, impatient, impulsive, and, before collapse reaches her, priding herself on the multiplicity of duties she can at one and the same time perform, an accomplishment by no means a virtue, as this broad sweep of labor ultimately results in collapse.

Prominent among the many causes for the defect called leanness, are nervous worriment, too little fresh air, and mal-assimilation, which may be due to one or the other or both the preceding. These may give rise to organic weaknesses, which in many cases grow into grave conditions before medical aid is sought; or they may be the result of organic weakness. In extreme cases, absolute rest, fresh air in plenty, simple, frequent feeding, and massage are the beginning treatment for home cases, whatever may be the cause.

By absolute rest, I mean that the patient must be isolated from all care or knowledge of care. Not even the interesting phases of home life should reach her. A quiet, sunny room, and a cheerful, but not talkative, attendant are the chief characteristics of this home rest cure. This will seem an impossibility to the woman who is able to go about her usual routine; but if she will but recall that her real duty is to restore and preserve her health, and so spare her friends the calamity of constantly caring for her in her invalidism, she will find it easily possible. Two months' isolation in a room of her own home should appeal to her as a more desirable issue than as many years in an institution, the fate that is sure to be hers if she neglects these early warnings. She must move out of herself, and allow Nature opportunity to restore her worn-out body.

By simple, frequent feeding, I refer to the milk dietary prescribed by our specialists. These methods should be carefully studied, and the use of heavier foods added, according to the conditions of the patient.

Massage should be mainly for limbs and back, unless the physician's diagnosis decides the advisability of it for viscera. Except in some cases of uterine weakness, massage for the digestive viscera will be of great value.

The foregoing remarks apply to those cases where emaciation is the result or accompaniment of some serious organic disease, or where it is the result of mal-nutrition or dyspepsia. In all such cases the dietary is matter for careful individual study, and only the most general principles of diet can be made universally applicable. Rest, food, fresh air, and massage, however, will always apply.

In average cases of leanness, where no especial disease exists, a few simple rules carefully observed will be of great advantage in improving weight.

Plenty of sleep and fresh air; avoidance of worry; repose of manner; daily cold bathing (see chapter on Bathing); absolute rest, from a half hour to two hours, after the noon meal; frequent, easily-digested meals, gradually increasing in quantity; and massage and exercise to improve tissue growth, constitute the thin woman's curriculum.

The exercise prescribed in the foregoing chapters will serve for bringing tissue change.

Milk and cream should enter largely into the dietary. In case it causes acidity, a little salt or bicarbonate of soda, or both, may be added. Matzoon is a valuable aid in tissue building.* Eggs, game, fish, mutton, bread

* Matzoon is a predigested food made from sterilized milk, and according to Prof. William H. Porter, M.D., in an article

and plenty of butter, cod-liver oil, baked apples, soups of marrow bones, vegetables, and other nourishing, easily digested foods of this order, had best form the staples of dietary. Grapes and oranges, pears, peaches, plums, apricots (cooked or uncooked), and other large fruits, except bananas, are valuable foods.

I refrain from any more specific remarks on this subject, however, as nearly every case comes within the province of the physician, and the instructor in physical culture should act only in concert with him. No two cases of this kind present conditions of sufficient similarity for the establishment of general rules. Nearly every case can be improved by systematic, carefully prescribed exercise; but the prescription should be specific, and not general. The general character of the exercises from which the prescriptions should be made is shown in the lesson of Recumbent Posture Movements.

---

in Merck's Bulletin, vol. vi. Nos. 1 and 2, it contains fully double the amount of nourishment found in koumyss. It is very smooth and palatable, and is strongly endorsed by leading physicians. Its originator is Dr. Dadirrian, a naturalized Armenian. His laboratory is at 73 Lexington Avenue, New York.

CHAPTER XXIV

FATIGUE AND REST

" Rest is the sweet sauce of labor."—PLUTARCH.

THE necessity of analyzing the sensation we call fatigue, and the theory of rest has come to the notice of but few of us, even those whose lives of care demand a rational comprehension of these subjects. Fatigue has seemed an inevitable condition of our hurried lives; and rest, nature's antidote, sparingly administered, and usually dispensed with as soon as the top of the hill is sighted. When the abilities thus overtaxed are exhausted, collapse is the result, and the rest cure yawns to receive the victim. What a blessing that we have those retreats, although they are but almshouses for impoverished humanity of good degree!

Exercise of any kind involves brain, spinal cord, and nerves; and overwork, either of mind or muscle, affects the individual unfavorably.

La Grange, in his "Physiology of Bodily Exercise," describes physical fatigue as "the sensation experienced by the individual after excessive muscular activity. It is a true regulator of work, which becomes the more sensitive the greater the danger which the exercise is causing the organism.

"In a feeble man, the sensation of fatigue is very painful, as the organs have less resistance, consequently undergo more easily damages due to fatigue."

He explains repose as "the necessary interval for the power of repair possessed by living organism as the essential condition for the elimination of the waste products of work; or the period necessary for the blood current to wash out the muscle and carry away waste products which are loading its fibres.

"Muscular work causes exaggeration of vital phenomena, and gives to all the functions a greater intensity; it quickens the pulse and respiration, and raises the temperature of the body. Rest slows the pulse and respiration, and lowers the temperature of the body."

Mental fatigue is less easily defined than physical fatigue. It is recognized in every home. Its synonyms are legion. More seriously than physical fatigue it threatens our country with dire disaster. We may classify it in three stages. First, nervousness, or Americanitis as foreigners call it; second, nervous exhaustion; third, nervous prostration. In its first stage, it may be easily overcome by adopting rational living habits. The second stage presages danger; but if organic conditions are favorable, and ample time allowed for a complete recovery, a useful life may yet result. The third stage stamps the victim an invalid, and she and her friends are fortunate, indeed, if comfort ever comes to her. Possibly, she may suffer little or no pain, but an indescribable feeling of exhaustion and irritability that is rarely overcome attends this condition. We speak of this state as neurasthenia; and while it is visited upon many business men, it is deplorably the fate of American women. It is doubtless due in most cases to faulty nutrition and insufficient rest. Nerves properly fed, used, and rested do not complain. They are long suffering, but rebel at continued imposition, and collapse is the result. Enfeebled digestion, lack of assimilation, imperfect circulation, mark the neurasthenic patient.

Everybody should understand himself sufficiently to keep within his limit of comfortable existence. Exhaustion should never be experienced. When a person finds that one hour's work of any certain kind brings fatigue, he should keep the recurrence of that duty within a fifty-minute limit next time, providing the conditions remain the same. We seldom find an American heeding the danger point or danger signals.

Mental fatigue may often be relieved by changing the subject of thought, even when no physical aid is brought to bear upon it; but the influence best calculated to rest the tired mind is bodily exercise, arranged to draw the excess of blood from brain to muscle, and accompanied by respiratory exercises to reoxygenate the blood. By this plan the mind may be kept in a wholesome condition.

For this practice I recommend something as follows:

FOOT MOVEMENT.—Neck firm; *heels raise.* (10 repetitions.) Be careful to maintain good posture.

SHOULDER-BLADE MOVEMENT.—*Arm stretching* or *circling.* (12 repetitions.) Careful to practice slowly and resistively.

TRUNK MOVEMENT.—Neck firm; *trunk bend* or *twist*. (5 repetitions.)

RESPIRATORY MOVEMENT.—*Arms sideways raise, inhaling*. (10 repetitions.)

Close with the beginning foot movement.

The movements are described in the preceding lessons.

This occupies but five minutes, and if practiced in a draught of fresh air, and from good posture, it will prove a mine of advantage.

Too long-continued concentration of will power on exercise of any one kind fatigues. In such instances rest is often experienced by a change of exercise. It may even be exertion of a more wearying nature than that which produced the fatigue, but it is sure to direct energy to other groups of muscles, allowing a fresh current of blood to circulate through those overtaxed, nourishing and resting them.

For example: writing, or other hand exercise that employs the flexor muscles, causes fatigue that can be dissipated by a hand extension movement; *i. e.*, opening the hand slowly and forcibly by contracting the muscles on the outer side. It is a mistake to clench the hand in gymnastic exercise for this purpose. Labor has already overforced the flexor muscles, and we must isolate these and energize the extensors. (See lesson on Recumbent Posture Movements.) Arm flexors are rested by shoulder-blade movements, and chest raising is sure to be restful after long-continued sitting occupation, with chest drooped. Fatigue from walking or bicycle riding may be relieved by assuming recumbent posture, neck firm, and practicing a slow bending and stretching of the ankles. The movement from this posture rests the muscles, even though the same ones are employed that have become fatigued; less energy is required than if erect posture were maintained, and the venous current is accelerated by both the position and movement. Twenty successive repetitions of this movement, followed by ten minutes or more of repose, with feet resting on a plane higher than the trunk (posture LXVIII., Recumbent Movements), will bring good results.

Rapid exertion, like running for a street car, should be avoided by those unaccustomed to violent exercise. A woman will sometimes not regain in several hours the vigor expended in such unnecessary haste. Far better lose that car, or even miss a train, than deplete the health by an injudicious outlay of energy and strength. A rapid walk is not apt to fatigue a woman of good vital health, if the speed is gradually accelerated. In the act of walking, the body is constantly supported, the balance changing easily from heel to toe. But in running, there is an instant between steps when the body is in complete suspension, having no support, and more energy is expended in throwing the weight thus from step to step than would be used in rapid walking. When it is necessary to run, the pace should be gradually increased from a walk, the head should be held erect, the chest raised, and comfortable breathing through the nose maintained. The run should not end abruptly, but should gradually merge into the rapid walk, and this into the normal pace. Treat yourself as you would a valuable horse, in regard to speed.

Running up stairs is not only bad for the health, but is also undignified and ungraceful; yet many women persist in doing it, to their harm. I have explained the theory of fatigue from running; add to that the resistance offered by raising the weight of the body from stair to stair, and you will see clearly why it is an unhygienic custom. The task of climbing stairs need not be a fatiguing one, if properly executed. The trunk should be held erect and the chest should not be allowed to droop. Place the foot flat on the stair, and steadily raise the body from this support (posture XCVI.). The knee-stretch movement is here particularly demonstrated. Advance steadily; do not pause between steps, as momentum is thus lost, and additional energy is needed to advance the next step.

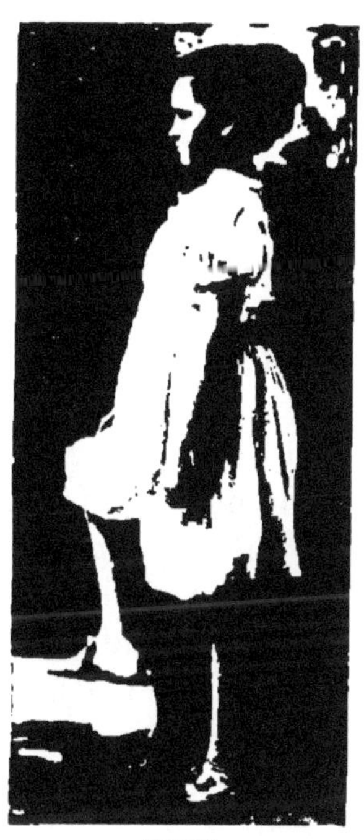

XCVI.

Often what we call fatigue is really hunger. The nourishment of our last meal has already been entirely used up, and the blood needs a fresh supply to use in running the human engine. It is necessary to satisfy this demand by some simple, easily assimilated food. A cup of warm broth, clam juice, gruel, milk, or matzoon, an egg taken raw, a baked apple, a slice of well-buttered whole-wheat bread, or some other nourishing food should be taken. Such refreshment, while it answers the demand, does not tax the digestive powers sufficiently to render continuance of work a harmful proceeding.

If Americans would but interpret correctly the word "economy," fatigue would not be so constant an attendant on their lives. In the majority of homes, economy is applied only in reference to finance. It has no definition in regard to the expenditure of physical and mental resources. Economy of time is only a trifle more intelligently dealt with. A woman fancies she is saving time when she employs her mind and her hands on different subjects at one and the same time. She wonders why the making of a cake tires her while the cook would experience no fatigue under the same amount of labor. The solution would be easy, if she would but realize that the cook's mind does not reach out to other subjects while engaged in that occupation; but her own is grasping after a score of other duties and claims, wholly foreign to what she is engaged in. With that cake she stirs the entire day's programme, plans her next season's wardrobe, arranges the education of the children, the charity work in the church, and attends to a score more of duties and interests ; hence her fatigue. Hands can follow brain dictation, but tire if working at odds with the brain. When hands are active, try and concentrate the mind on their occupation. When the brain is working in the abstract, relax muscular force. The energies are thus conserved, and better work results.

Much energy is wasted by unnecessarily holding one's self in a tense muscular condition. This tension is equally harmful whether one is under influence of physical pain or mental stress.

We can bear pain more easily by relaxing the muscles than by tightening them. The clenched hands and suspended breath, when one is in the dentist's chair, increase the suffering. Of course we must have a certain amount of courage to meet suffering and danger; but true strength is wasted, not increased, by the exaggerated force we mistake as helpful. Even the schoolgirl resorts to tension, and endeavors to concentrate her thoughts by twisting her foot around the chair-leg, pushing her tongue into the roof of her mouth, and forcing her muscles to rigidity when they should be in repose. The restless tapping of the fingers or foot, the strained attitude of attention at concert or church, as if endeavoring to aid the performer or speaker, or the earnest efforts at helping the carriage horses when haste is especially necessary—all are a useless drain upon vital energy, which should be avoided.

A certain amount of repose maintained in every act of life will help to preserve the energies. Repose in walking and in standing is acquired by proper, systematic exercise. Let the chair, carriage, or couch, as the case may be, hold your physical weight; do not hold yourself up on either. Particularly on retiring should the muscles be relaxed. Sleep is the more easily induced if we make ourselves conscious of physical weight, and feel that every limb is resting heavily upon the couch. The mind is often hard to relax; we can help this along by moving out of the physical body, and by letting the mind wander untrammelled. Do not try to stop thinking, and especially do not burden the mind with such wrongly prescribed remedies as adding imaginary columns of figures, counting sheep, etc. It takes a vigorous person to induce sleep by any such means, and I have yet to find a person of weak nerves who has been able to benefit by this unnecessary exercise of will power. Let the mind alone. It cannot run riot long if we simply do not try to chain or control it. A few simple exercises arranged to draw the blood to the extremities, and a simple respiratory exercise (see lesson on Recumbent Posture Movements), will usually rest the overburdened mind, and sleep will prove a sweet restorer.

Cares often burden the mind after sleep comes. This generally indicates an unhealthy physical condition, although it may be entirely due to mental fatigue. (For children's dreams see chapter on Early Life and Training of Children.)

The American voice is apt to be very tiring. It is in most cases sharp or shrill, loud, harsh, or guttural—the exception is one of smooth-flowing tones—and both speaker and listener are consequently fatigued. Why is it that so much attention is given to educating the mind, while the voice is so wofully neglected? Unless a girl gives promise of being a *prima donna*, money is rarely expended in cultivating her voice, even though it might prove her most lasting charm. Nothing soothes a sick, a nervous, or even an angry person so much as a sweet, well-modulated voice; and a harsh one is as irritating as discordant music to the nerves. Especially should a mother, nurse, teacher, minister, or doctor have an even, well-governed voice. A child with a tendency to St. Vitus's dance should never be allowed to hear a sharp or an impatient tone. Women who are subject to bad tempers will find much help to self-control through calming the voice, and making the respiration slower. Oblige an angry child to breathe slowly and talk gently, and immediately his anger will soften. Impatience and repining wear terribly on nerve vigor, and inscribe themselves upon the face in ugly lines and wrinkles.

Fear is also very exhaustive; and could we but fortify ourselves against that emotion, the heart would have much less hard work to perform. You can easily verify this by noting the heart-beat of a delicate child, or of a timid animal, after being subjected to fright. On the other hand, fear is frequently a stimulant to fatigued muscles; so also is pleasure. For illustration, a tired army may be incited to untold energy by sudden tidings of a victory, and also by news of defeat when retreat is ordered. A child can always be stimulated to exertion by the anticipation of pleasure. Fear, not joy, however, is producing Americanitis.

Fear and rivalry, and we might also add despondency, are co-workers to the ruin of peace and happiness. If we could but see the humorous side of despondencies, for there always is a humorous side, how much suffering we could spare ourselves!

It is often hard to determine between fatigue and indolence, in the case of a child, and one in charge of children should study well their physical conditions before deciding. Never compare one child's strength with another's, nor one woman's strength with another's; each must be estimated according to her individual resources and idiosyncrasies.

Every woman of delicate physique should take a half hour's repose in the middle of each day; after the noon meal is a good hour for this. It economizes in labor and time, as she is better fitted to perform her duties afterward. I don't mean she should lie down and read, but compose herself, and allow her body complete rest, free from mental as well as physical effort. Even ten minutes of such entire repose gives much benefit.

A woman while entertaining callers should make herself and her guests as comfortable as possible. When a guest rises to depart, the hostess should consider the visit completed, and not prolong the conversation unless the visitor will be seated again. This is not only courteous, but spares both guest and hostess painful fatigue.

Strength is often needlessly exhausted by dwelling on mental and physical sufferings. It is most unwholesome to rehearse ills, even to one's best friends; it is unwholesome for both parties. Better put the best foot forward, and make the best of life, confiding ailments only to one's physician, or to some one able to lend strength or courage. Mere emotional sympathy is harmful.

It is unwise to grovel in other people's misery. Lend a helping hand to the depressed, but do not let your strength go out in imagining yourself in his place. The text, " Bear ye one another's burdens," does not necessarily include assuming his misery. Sentimentality is not of advantage in charity work. Work practically among the distressed, make them comfortable as far as is rationally practicable, but save your best energies to brighten your own home. Many noble charity workers mistake their real duty by exhausting themselves with emotional work among the poor, thus robbing their home circle of the genial companionship they owe there.

In case of illness in the family, fortify your strength for emergencies, by sufficient nourishment and rest. Do not allow your appetite to flag with that of the sick one. This you may think is more easily said than done; but it should be easily done, since husbanding your strength may enable you to actually save the life of your loved one. Take a practical view, and put aside the emotional. It can be done if you view it rationally. If your throat is too contracted from grief to admit the passage of solid food, drink nourishing broths instead, and nature will help you in regaining your courage. Do not so far mistake duty as to sacrifice your life to save another's. Study, instead, to save both. Let your head rule your emotions, and always practice economy of energy. A cool, practical hand may save a life; and a lifetime of ill-health may be caused by indulging in ill-judged emotions and unnecessary efforts made from mistaken ideas of duty.

Every woman, and especially every girl, should be kept free from fictitious emotional excitement. It renders girls morbid, and dulls their capacity for real sentiment, to allow them to indulge in emotional love, even for one another. Abnormal emotions often embitter a woman's whole life; and the emotional love of a child for a playmate, a dog, or some other pet is often unwholesome in many ways. The desire for such habits will vanish under proper influences. The best antidote for this is well-regulated gymnastic exercise and fresh-air sports, with no time allowed for moping or dreaming.

Misdirected duty, impulsive outlay of strength, unskilled labor, the grasping for the unattainable, social and financial rivalry—these, not the real duties of life, wear our women out.

Nagging worriments of life are more wearing than real burdens. Don't admit a nagging person (even if it is your mother-in-law) to enter into your life. If she must dwell under your roof, have a clear and definite understanding as to any bone of contention, settle it calmly and kindly, and let it be clearly understood as then settled, and that no subsequent nagging will be permitted. A person thus armed can win any battle.

Financial slavery is the curse of many valuable lives. A proud woman cannot endure the slavery her husband, lavish in every other direction, sometimes places her under in the matter of money.

A capable woman worker, performing well the duties of a man in a similar position, chafes under the galling fact that she receives but half the wages which would be paid the man.

The laws of physical culture are the laws of nature. We study her demands—the theory of cause and effect, the human body as a machine, the mind as the individual—and readjust these laws through her means where we find they have been ignored.

One of nature's greatest lessons is rest, repose. I do not use the word "repose" as a synonym for "deënergizing the system," a phrase made ridiculous by the caricaturing Delsarte's beautiful work has suffered at the hands of so many incompetents, but as the best that nature can give us. Rest! The cessation from toil that nature always demands; the freedom from a worrying existence; peace, if the term please us better.

CHAPTER XXV

BICYCLING

"Venture not to the utmost bounds of even lawful pleasure; the limits of good and evil join."—FULLER.

THE bicycle is a boon to over-burdened Americans, and is destined to prove woman's emancipation from the slavery of dress.

Those advanced in years, as well as those still in the enjoyment of youth, appreciate the pleasure of this pastime, which combines the exhilaration of the exercise and rapid motion with the good effects of fresh air.

Business men and women and tired mothers alike need an encouraging influence to take them into the open air, and for this, and the other advantages here suggested, we have great reason to appreciate the bicycle.

As with any other valuable adjunct to pleasure, we must, while studying its advantages, also give ear to its disadvantages, and, in adapting its use, make sure to avoid attendant errors.

That the recreation is often carried to excess, and that bad posture is a criminal offence not only to the figure and health of the rider, but also to the eye of the beholder, are truths daily forced upon us, and no space is necessary here for advice that would be but repetitious. There are graver features of harm to result from the indiscriminate use of the wheel. I will suggest a few, but lack of space will prevent my elaborating on any of them.

In all specific exercises, certain muscles are developed at the expense of others; and the bicycle devotee, as well as the professional oarsman, cannot remain symmetrical in muscular development without the aid of other exercises adapted to strengthen the muscles not actively employed in these sports. Rowing develops the abdominal muscles, and those of the back, forearm, wrist, and front of the leg. The chest becomes narrow, the biceps small, and the shoulders more or less drooping. In order, therefore, to make rowing beneficial, the oarsman should also use exercises to direct the energies to the groups of muscles that oppose or antagonize the ones over-forced. The tennis player also suffers from unequal use of the energies; and the skill of the croquet player is still more unfavorably employed, as drooping chest posture is added to one-sided exercise.

In bicycling, the energy is directed to certain groups of muscles, while others are merely placed on a continuous stretch, which is not exercise, and still others are neglected altogether. Among those unemployed are the chest muscles and intercostals, which should be our most flexible ones for advantage in good respiration, and also as an aid in resistance to disease, especially of lungs. It has been proved that weak lungs have been strengthened under moderate use of the wheel, but the benefit has come from the fresh air, rapid motion, and the pleasure afforded, rather than from the exercise.

The muscles specifically involved in bicycling depend upon the pace, the grade of the track, the posture assumed, and the repose and skill (or lack of it) possessed by the rider. The slow or walking pace uses primarily the muscles of the calf and thigh, and, after skill in poise is attained, places no more demand on trunk muscles than ordinary walking does. In other words, after one has learned to ride, the pastime ceases to be a specific exercise.

In propelling the bicycle up a grade, or in speeding, especially when the trunk is inclined forward, the muscles of the back, arms, shoulder-blades, and even abdomen are called into heavy use by being placed on a tension. This tension, however, is not of value in rendering the muscles flexible and capable of good contractility, essentials necessary in preserving the powers of the body. The blood current is called to the muscles wherein the energy is localized, but tissue growth and destruction do not take place as they do from exercises that are attended with momentary pauses of relaxation, and that force the blood current to different groups of muscles in succession or order, rather than placing so many on a stretch at once, and consequently making so heavy a demand upon the circulatory apparatus.

The height of the handle-bar and of the seat are also matters of important consideration. The individual's length of arms and height of trunk, not entire stature, should be considered in deciding these. Short arms need a higher handle-bar than longer ones do, and the person whose length is in favor of trunk rather than legs, needs the higher handles.

Women generally need higher handle-bars

than men do. The distance from seat to pedals should also be adjusted in accord with the leg measurement. The heel should not be unduly raised, nor should it be depressed, in the leg extension and flexion attendant upon the exercise. The height of the saddle regulates this. Economy of strength is gained through having these mechanical adjustments accurate. The most harmful feature of riding is the pressure of the narrow saddle. The narrow saddle causes pressure upon the pelvic organs, especially if the "scorching" position is assumed, and is exceedingly harmful, affecting both sexes unfavorably. Some say with indifference, "Yes, the narrow saddle causes discomfort, but one gets used to it." "Getting used to it" means, in many cases, permanent injury. The ideal saddle is yet to be found, although it is hoped that the recent improvements will tend greatly toward preventing the injuries to nerve health that in some cases have proved alarming. The "Duplex" seems to be the most favorable to the health of the rider.

The exercise of the lower limbs to the neglect of the upper muscles, combined with the continued leverage brought to bear on the hips, directs an excess of blood current to the muscles and organs of that part of the body, which is of itself pernicious. These two, the saddle pressure on the pelvic organs and the leg exercise, combine to cause a nervous irritation which will wreck the health and future career of many a valuable life, if strict measures are not adopted to prevent their continuance. Let mothers look well into this from an anatomical and physiological standpoint, before allowing their children's future to be wrecked by a pastime that can easily be supplemented so as to make it a healthful rather than baleful exercise.

The "bicycle face" is generally understood to be the external expression of fear and anxiety; but whether it is from such a cause, or the result of nerve pressure above alluded to, it is certainly necessary to take measures to prevent it by better preparation in skill and poise, if the cause lies in their lack, or in adopting a saddle and assuming a posture that can cause no irritation to sensitive nerves.

Those of hemorrhoidal tendencies are apt to suffer irritation from wheeling, and pelvic weaknesses are liable to be seriously increased by the exercise.

Dress is of engrossing interest to our women riders. It must be comfortable, artistic, womanly. (For undergarments I refer to the chapter on Dress). The knickerbockers and leggings should be the same color as the skirt; clinging material should not be used in the skirt; use, instead, stiff material, as brilliantine, so that the leg motion is not noticeable. The skirt should reach below the knee, so that in walking it is perfectly in keeping with the womanly tastes of the present age. It should also be so adjusted as to hang gracefully over the wheel. Jacket and cap need not suggest masculinity.*

Symmetry of growth and stature, apportionate use of the muscles, and flexibility of muscles, especially of chest walls, cannot be obtained through bicycling alone, and in a few years the need of supplementary exercises will be generally felt, as it already is in many cases.

The great needs in this are balance, arm, chest, shoulder-blade and lateral trunk movements. I will give here a formula, and would suggest that the lessons in the foregoing chap-

* Mrs. Rew's "Delsarte Ideal Bicycle Costume" appeals to the business woman and schoolgirl, as well as to the wheelwoman. Its artistic, as well as hygienic, cut of waist and skirt, and the attachment of knickerbockers against the skirt, are salient points characteristic of this suit.

ter be adapted to it, repeating the movements as indicated in the formula from the same lessons.

PREPARATORY EXERCISE FOR BICYCLING.

Respiratory Movement.
Head Movement.
Balance Movement.
Shoulder-blade Movement.
Chest Movement.
Balance Movement.
Back Movement.
Abdominal Movement.
Shoulder-blade Movement.
Lateral Trunk Movement.
Balance Movement.
Respiratory Movement.

The lesson of Recumbent Posture Movements should be practiced after returning from a fatiguing ride. By exercising the muscles, even the tired ones, from restful posture, the blood is forced through the tissues without causing strain, and great advantage results from washing out the muscle fibres with a fresh blood current, and thereby relieving congestion. If but little time is allowed for rest exercise, let the formula cover (from Recumbent Posture lesson) the following:

Chest Raising.

Foot Movement.

Abdominal Movement (hook-lying, hips raise).

Respiratory Movement, from posture LXVIII.

CHAPTER XXVI

DRESS: ITS INFLUENCE ON MIND AND ON HEALTH

"Fine clothes are stilts to individuality."—BRINTON.

"It is the mind that dresses the body."—MULFORD.

AN able thinker has said, "The human person is composed of three parts: body, soul, and dress."

The inference to be drawn is, that dress is a more powerful factor in the creation of the individual than we have heretofore acknowledged.

We all feel our best when dressed our best.

The clothes we wear exert great influence on the conception and execution of our ideas and aims, both from a physiological and an æsthetic standpoint. Æsthetically considered, dress is an exponent of character. It also, to a great extent, shapes character. Prentice Mulford, in his "Religion of Dress," explains clearly this reflex influence.

The slovenly mind is expressed in slovenly

attire. Improve the dress, and the mind will show like improvement. The habitually well-dressed individual will suffer in moral tone if forced to appear in uncleanly or mean clothing. For every age and every grade of society we find mind and dress reciprocal influences.

We need to live amid plenty of color and light, and it will be a boon to humanity when black drapery as an emblem of mourning is reckoned among the customs of the past. The bereaved would find comfort and peace the sooner were she to attire herself in soft gray, écru, or cream tints, instead of black, whether she be of a practical or an emotional nature; and thus attired she would carry with her an air of calmness which would make her presence welcome everywhere. In contrast with such influence, her emblems of grief cast a gloom over all natures with whom she comes in contact, and her health and the health of others suffer in consequence.

A woman should study her figure and her complexion in arranging texture and color for dress. Eyes and hair give suggestions of color theme in nature's plan, which should be studied for individual dress. Tints must harmonize, else mental discord is sure to follow.

Age should also be considered. While the elderly woman appears a caricature when dressed in girlish attire, we regret still more to see any woman dressed "too old" for her years. Woman's age is as she heralds it; and we deplore the woman who labels herself old. Let the elderly woman dress as the middle-aged, the middle-aged as the young woman, and then we will have no old women.

Dress should always be suited to climatic conditions. A cold, raw day calls for warm tints, and a hot day for cool tints. The woman who intentionally overdoes elaborateness on a plain occasion, shows lack of refinement.

The physiological influence dress has on our lives, necessarily claims most space in this chapter.

Our women lack the fullest expansion of their abilities, from enslavement to custom, and the most arbitrary of custom's rules are in relation to dress. From the tight glove and the narrow-toe shoe to the lace veil, freedom is curbed and ambitions are checked by these barriers. But it is underwear rather than outside clothing that especially hampers good growth and activity.

In this chapter I mean only to suggest plans

for the adjustment of clothing, to secure economy of health, prevention of invalidism, and exaltation of the individual.

Clothing to be worn next the skin should be adapted to facilitate its functions, and selected with that end in view. None should be allowed which may chafe, irritate, or chill it. The skin is not generally valued at its true worth, nor do we realize how intimate is the relation between its healthy action and the true happiness of the individual. Too often it is considered a mere covering for softer tissues beneath. It serves us for this purpose, but for much more besides. The skin is one of the most important sewers of the body. Its perspiratory pores are very numerous—twenty-five hundred to the square inch, two million three hundred thousand in all. If straightened out and placed end to end they would extend over two and a half miles in length.

These pores open outward from the glands that secrete impurities thrown off by the blood in its circulation, and exude an average of two pounds for the adult during twenty-four hours. I will take no more space, however, for anatomical data, except to suggest the subject as one for broader research.

I quote these facts merely to show the need of properly clothing the body, if for no other reason than to protect the skin for the preservation of its functions. It is obviously necessary that the body be clothed with material of a porous nature, so that air may reach the skin. It is necessary also that it be clothed evenly, not overburdened in some parts, to their detriment, from overheating, and excluding the action of the air; nor neglected in others, to their detriment, by chilling the surface, causing congestion, or colds as we say. Experience teaches that wool is lighter, more agreeable to the touch, and a better protection both winter and summer, than any other material used for underclothing. Our women are apt to denounce wool from prejudice, unmindful of the fact that our manufacturers now have the daintiest and softest of textures in this fabric—textures that would be admired were they prepared for outer rather than under wear. From prejudice many also say that the wool garment for the lower limbs would overheat them, utterly disregarding the fact that the waist and lower chest are overheated by the use of air-tight clothing that custom has for many generations beguiled us into wearing. I dislike to feel that our women are inconsistent, but in no other way can I see this trait so strongly marked as in this of underwear.

In this chapter I shall make but a few suggestions, trusting that they will help many toward the initiatory steps in freedom of dress.

The union suit, in place of the two garments of former custom, is a valued innovation in woman's wardrobe. It spares much inconvenience of bulk around the waist and hips ; and, if properly laundered, shrinkage need not result, provided, of course, good material is purchased.

The union suit for winter should reach the ankle, as well as wrist. Much rheumatism, neuralgia, and other ills would be spared our women were they to observe this caution as carefully as they do the style of outer clothing.*

* In urging this style of underwear, I will say that the Ypsilanti (Mich.) Health Underwear Co. furnish the most satisfactory garments, inasmuch as they have every variety of fabrics, from the daintiest to the heaviest, in colors to suit different tastes, and in desirable combinations of neck shape, and sleeve and leg lengths. They also weave goods to order, in case one's figure is other than normal. If their printed directions are followed in laundering, very little shrinkage is noticed. I give the experience of many years' trial, and I feel the information is valuable in helping women in their selection of goods.

The knit abdominal band is a valuable garment for children, and also for adults who are inclined to weakness of abdominal organs. Difficulty will be experienced in keeping it down in place unless it is shaped to the hips by cutting it (two to four inches) upward at the hips. For children's wear it may also be necessary to have a shoulder-strap to keep it in place.

Stockings should be adjusted after the union suit is on. Equestrian tights, which are worn outside the stockings, will hold the latter in place with no other support. In case the tights are worn to the knee only, instead of to the ankle, a safety pin may be used, if desired, fastening the stocking top, union suit, and tights together. This is necessary only for the peace of mind of the wearer, who has been accustomed to the old-time methods of hose support, and feels that the new methods would be insufficient. A skirt of light weight, and of color corresponding as closely as possible with the dress, completes the underclothing of the lower limbs.

This plan is far better than the old-time idea of numerous skirts, inasmuch as the back is relieved of the weight of clothing, the waist of the multiplicity of bands, and the lower limbs of impediments in walking. Besides, the members are better protected from cold and dampness when each is clothed singly in a closely fitting garment, instead of the skirt drapery of former years.

Boots should be of thick but flexible material, firm but pliable sole, with insole of corrugated felt, to absorb perspiration. They should, when purchased, fit the feet, with no need of the breaking-in process. The heel should be no higher than to give sufficient height to the natural arch of the foot. A well-poised body rests alike on both feet, the heel and ball of each foot together supporting the weight. The high heel, even though it may be but one lift too high, throws the body forward in a way not only to prevent good poise, but often to cause fatigue or weakness of back at waist.

The pointed toe should not be worn, even though the foot has for years been trained to this shape. It prevents good circulation, and frequently causes bunions. Repose of posture and ease in walking are impossible if freedom of the toes is denied.

Care should be taken that the feet are kept warm, as well as dry. In case a change in weather finds one unprepared for severer influences, a cold may be prevented by placing several folds of paper—blotting-paper is preferred—inside the shoes, protecting particularly the hollow of the foot.

Felt slippers or shoes are excellent for house wear; they afford better protection and give better support than the softer sole, knit slipper, and, on account of their porosity, are fully as hygienic. Some shoe of this description should form part of every woman's and girl's wardrobe, and should be kept easily at hand. Many a cold or set-back in convalescence would be spared were this observed, and the thoughtless custom avoided of stepping from the warm bed to the floor, with the feet unprotected.

The corset is an all-absorbing topic among women. We may almost consider that the arguments for and against its use have established partisan antagonism. Devotees would as soon allow criticism against their honesty as against their corsets; while equally strong discussion arises from artists and health seekers. Artists deplore its destructive influence on beauty. The truths of the health-seeker have been sounded in every land, hence I will not repeat them. Its history and the wrongs attending its use should be rationally set forth, but not as unexplained maledictions that tend to antagonize rather than convert the corset wearer, as is too often the case.

Mrs. Helen Gilbert Ecob has written a clever book, entitled "The Well Dressed Woman," in which, among other good things, she gives in detail the history of the corset. It is a pleasing genealogy, one that women should claim the privilege of reading. Mrs. Ecob certainly proves that the corset never was an emblem of strength, physically, mentally, or morally.

We will leave history, and consider nineteenth century facts. The corset causes confusion and discord in the grandest of all creations—the human body. A woman or girl is not mentally her best when inconvenienced by physical discomfort of any kind, and stiff or tight waist clothing is a great source of inconvenience, affecting some more seriously than others, and earlier in life. It interferes with one's comfort. It destroys one's grace and ease. It checks good circulation, and thereby hastens development of weak tendencies and of superfluous adipose, which should rank with rheumatism and other diseases as a strong symptom of unnatural conditions. Girls break down and women wear out under the rule of the corset. So closely are some women wedded to their corsets that on recovering from illness they boast, not that they are on their feet again, but that they are once more in their corsets.

I will make no concession to wearing it comfortably. That may be possible while standing posture is maintained, but even the loose corset causes displacement of abdominal organs under change of posture, as sitting, stooping, climbing, stepping up stairs, etc. The physiological wrong of interrupting functions of lungs, heart, stomach, liver, and other internal organs, cannot fail to be apparent to every thinking mind, even though that individual desires to personally continue its use. She may be able to influence girls to dress more advantageously, even though she herself feels "too old to adopt new customs."

Let us consider the corset from an artistic and a moral standpoint.

Artistically, it interrupts a symmetrical plan, suggesting to the cultured mind amalgamation of several designs with no harmony of contour or proportion.

Morally, it teaches girls deception and artificiality. The mother does not mean her daughter to compress her waist, but still she sees it growing a trifle more narrow each week, until the girl is quite "shapely," as many mothers say. The girl has lost more than her natural proportions; she has lost the conception of the word "truth," by presenting an artificial figure to the world. We discountenance bleached hair and tinted cheeks, yet smile approvingly at artificial waists. No physical harm may result from use of hair bleach and rouge; merely the moral wrong of creating artificiality and deception in the individual mind; while these and also direst physical harm result from narrowing the waist.

For the women who for years have been accustomed to the support and warmth furnished by the corset I would recommend the health waist as a substitute, that being a garment easily laundered, and would urge that it be of as porous material as possible. The argument that it "doesn't fit" is a weak one; if women would seek as earnestly to find one that does fit them as they do for things they really want, they could easily find a desirable one. There is no longer lack of variety of style or texture. Manufacturers have learned that the stout, the thin, the tall, the short have an individuality of figure, and have well met the needs of each.

For the girl or for the woman young enough to restore her muscles and skin to normal vigor, I urge strongly that not even this waist be used. Wherein lies its need? Merely in the narrow idea of following custom. It cannot be needed for support, for firm, pliable, well-educated muscles hold the trunk in support always. It is not necessary for warmth, unless the tissues of the portion of the body referred to have been softened and weakened by the use of such a garment. It is not necessary for support of heavy petticoats, as these are to be supplanted by other garments.

A well-adjusted sleeveless dress form or lining, with hooks for attachment of the dress skirt, is convenient, and should always be worn unless the dress skirt and waist are in one piece. Dress skirts are no longer necessarily burdensome; light-weight fabrics, and these fastened to waists, are sure to give the freedom that passeth all understanding.

No clothing that has been or is to be worn during the day should be worn at night. Impurities are continually passing through the pores of the skin, and garments worn next to the body should be well aired at night for next day's use. A sleeveless undervest and a wool gown make the best night clothing for child, as well as adult. The fabric may be light or heavy, according to discretion. This mode of dressing the body makes chilling less probable when stepping from the warm bed into the cooler room, and also gives less need of heavy bed covers, hence sleep is more restful. If the wool gown is hung in the open air every day, there will be less frequent need of laundering than is the case with the cotton goods.

Disease germs thrive in foul air, and great care should be taken that good ventilation in wardrobes, shoe-closets, etc., is secured. The soiled clothes hamper should always stand in a well-ventilated place.

Economy is a necessary rule in most homes, but let us analyze the term well when applying it to clothing. To those who change about old-time customs, adopting undergarments recommended here, the original expenditure will, of course, be more than that of replenishing the former wardrobe; but this can be easily balanced by economy in laundry, as there will be fewer pieces to handle, and especially to mend and replenish. The tired hands that superintend the returned laundering will find peace through this great feature of emancipation, which means economy in time and in strength.

Tight gloves are another vexation to the physical soul, especially if that soul has a nucleus of gout or rheumatism in its extremities.

Veils injure the health of the nerves by forcing the sight through a confusing network placed between the eyes and the object toward which the vision is directed. If any one doubts this, better prove the remark by inducing a man to wear a lace veil all or part of a day, and then ask his opinion. Why should not women, as well as men, enjoy freedom for their eyes? Veils intensify certain colors, blend the artificial with the natural, and cover defects, but they also give evidence of the need of such an agent. Let the old and ugly cover their faces, if any one must. It is the privilege of the young, fresh face to prove the charm of reality.

My plea is only for the girls. If women choose to assert themselves too old to change habits of dress, I have no desire to argue against them; but let us rear our girls to their natural rights. Let us respect them as we do the boys. Let us dress them becomingly and fashionably, but, in doing this, let us arrange our American fashions to respect the mechanical and physiological laws of the body. Let us not profane the sacred temple, but, instead, harmonize the trio of created humanity—soul, body, dress.

CHAPTER XXVII

SYSTEMATIC BATHS

"So great is the effect of cleanliness upon man that it extends even to his moral character. Virtue never dwelt long with filth; nor do I believe there ever was a person scrupulously attentive to cleanliness who was a consummate villain." —RUMFORD.

THE anatomy of the skin is most interesting, and its physiology phenomenal, yet it receives less scientific thought and care than almost any other organ we possess.

The skin consists of three layers. The outer one is the epidermis, or cuticle, commonly called the scarf-skin; the next layer is the dermis, or true skin; and the inner layer is designated as the subcutaneous base on which the true skin rests.

The cuticle serves as a protection for the true skin. Its thickness varies on different parts of the body, and is greatest on the palms of the hands and soles of the feet.

The dermis includes two layers, the superficial papillary, and the deeper reticular layer.

The former consists of numerous highly sensitive eminences called papillæ. They are but one one-hundredth of an inch in length, and less than half that in diameter. They contain tiny nerve endings known as touch nerves. These organs of perception, besides aiding other senses on general matters of intelligence, give warning of heat, cold, injury, etc. They may be cultivated to an almost miraculous degree, as we often find them in the blind. The papillæ are distributed all over the body, but are most numerous on the palmar surfaces of hands and fingers. The cuticle is accurately moulded into the grooves between the papillæ, and serves as protection to these sensitive organs.

The reticular layer of the dermis is tough, flexible, and highly elastic. It protects the tissues underneath from violence. It consists of fibrous connective tissue, and fibrous elastic tissue, blood vessels, nerves, lymphatics, etc. Its meshes gradually coarsen as it approaches the base; globules of fat fill in the interstices.

The subcutaneous base, or third layer of skin, contains the perspiratory glands, sebaceous glands, and hair follicles; also the nutrient arteries, which form a network under

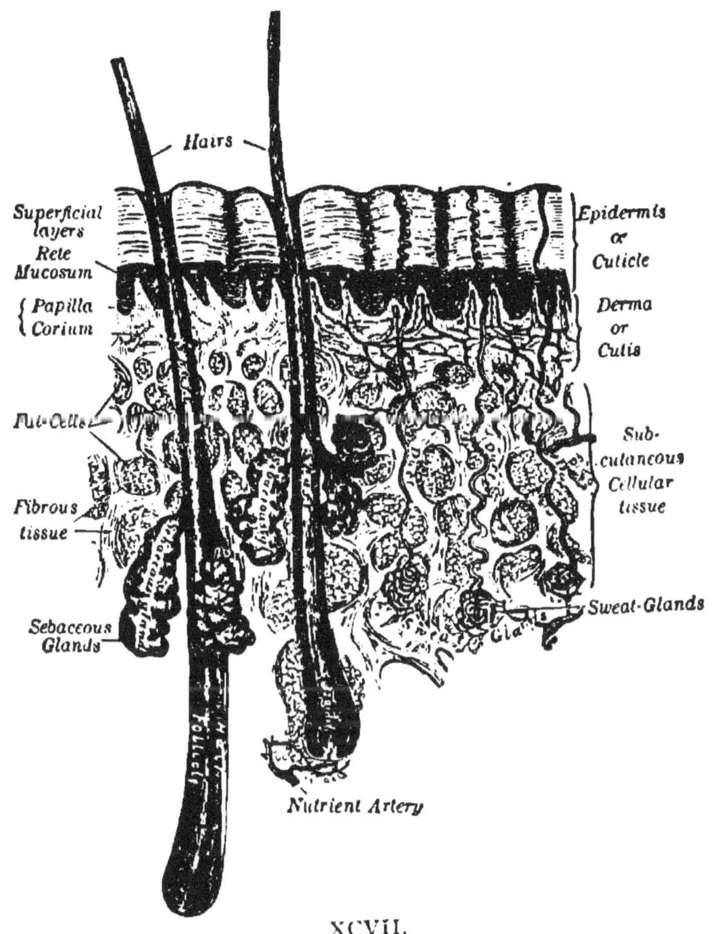
Hairs
Superficial layers
Rete Mucosum
Papilla
Corium
Fat-Cells
Fibrous tissue
Sebaceous Glands
Epidermis or Cuticle
Derma or Cutis
Sub-cutaneous Cellular tissue
Sweat-Glands
Nutrient Artery

XCVII.

the glands, and give off branches to supply them.

The skin has three uses, viz.: to regulate the temperature of the body, to protect the softer parts underneath, and to throw off effete matter from the perspiratory glands through the pores. The respiratory function of the skin is also an interesting and valuable study. The excretory function is especially promoted by the bath, and will, therefore, receive principal attention in this chapter.

The perspiratory glands are very numerous—two million three hundred thousand in the body. They are about one four-hundredth of an inch in diameter, and consist of a globular coil enveloped in a network of capillary vessels, the termination of the nutrient arteries. They serve as sewers of the system. Through their walls certain impurities are exuded from the blood, in form of perspiration. In its dry form it is known as insensible perspiration. Each gland opens spirally outward, through a duct which terminates in a pore. If straightened out, each would measure one-fifteenth of an inch; and added in length would average in the adult about two and a half miles of sewerage. During the twenty-four hours these throw off about two pounds of refuse matter.

The walls of these glands, tiny as they are, seem marvellously intelligent in their work. Each is independent in its activity, ceaselessly doing its share to purify the system, yet all working harmoniously, stimulated by muscular activity. Exercise is highly necessary in preserving the functions of the skin.

Great harm results from a burn or scald of much superficial extent, as the impurities which nature designed to eliminate through the pores are retained because of this functional interruption, and necessarily reabsorbed by the blood. Disease, the seriousness of which is in proportion to the extent of injury, results. In some cases death speedily ensues.

Continuous with the outer skin is that which lines the internal organs. The pores of this inner skin, or mucous membrane as it is called, resemble those of the outer in structure, and are the mediums through which the functions of the organs are performed.

Cleanliness is indeed akin to godliness, and there is nothing that lends more exaltation of spirit than the daily bath. In the days of Roman supremacy the bath was one of the most important features of life. The public baths were magnificently equipped, and everybody patronized them daily. The appointments for the rich were sumptuous in the extreme; and the poor were provided for at little or no expense. Perhaps we should not spend as much time daily as they did in the bath, but its importance cannot be overestimated. Bathing, like other hygienic expedients, should be rationally adjusted, and for this purpose every one should make a careful study of her own conditions, not comparing her strength to that of her more vigorous neighbor. Great and lasting harm often comes to a delicate woman from taking the cold shower or plunge bath upon the advice of a robust friend. A frail person, like a frail plant, cannot endure a severe "toughening process," but will thrive under suitable influences.

A thin-blooded, anæmic, neuralgic person, or one of light heart action, should avoid tub baths, even though carefully taken. When the entire body is simultaneously exposed to water, more blood is called to the surface than the internal organs can spare, the heart is overworked in attempts to supply the extra demand, and unfavorable reaction of some kind will sooner or later be experienced. With some it causes fainting; with others, chills; while still others experience fatigue, headache, or loss of appetite.

Evening is not a wise time for bathing, excepting partial baths for children, and is especially unsuitable for women. They are apt to have exhausted themselves during the day, and at night they need repose rather than the stimulating influence of the bath. The argument, "My night bath rests me," is frequently made. The explanation of this is, that it temporarily stimulates the papillæ; but it will sooner or later be attended by unfavorable results.

Sometimes years of imprudent bathing may not bring disaster to those of average health; but a time will come, even to them, when the system is in a receptive rather than a resistive condition, and nerve exhaustion or some other ills will be precipitated as a result of wrongs done the system by unhygienic bathing. Reaction from the night bath is intensified by the influences which sleep and the recumbent posture exert, and these combine to make it a most unhealthful custom. The night bath is also unnecessary so far as the functions of the skin are concerned, as the muscular exercise of the day should sufficiently stimulate the action of the pores.

Morning is the proper time for bathing. The night of repose does not encourage the elimination of effete matter through the skin, hence water is necessary for cleansing it. The bath also excites good circulation, and freshens the system, imbuing one with a feeling of self-respect imparted by nothing else. Let it be a daily habit for children, and in adult life it will have become second nature, and will act as a preventive of many physical ills, by increasing one's power of resistance.

I cannot better explain scientifically the beneficial effects of bathing than by quoting from Hare's "System of Practical Therapeutics," page 470, from the chapter by Dr. Simon Baruch, on "Effect of Peripheral Irritation on Tissue Metamorphosis."

"Ranke has enunciated the law that though the quantity of plasma and circulating albumen is constant, its production depends upon the quiescence or activity of the organs. He and Voit demonstrated that function is always connected with increased circulation in the organs, and that tissue change is coincident with circulating activity. As the blood is the chief carrier of material for tissue metamorphosis, it follows that any procedure by which the distribution of blood may be controlled must influence more or less the tissue changes. And when it is considered that temperature changes are either the cause or effect of tissue changes, any measures which control this important factor must aid in influencing tissue metamorphosis. That cold reduces and heat increases cell activity is axiomatic. But these are direct effects, which do not so frequently come within the therapeutic domain as the indirect results produced by reflex agencies, and which are paradoxically contrary to these. From the cautious experiments of Liebermeister, the fact has been deduced that oxidation, as ascertained by the excretion of CO_2, is enhanced by the external application of cold, and diminished by the external application of heat, so long as the body temperature is not disturbed. As soon as the body temperature is reduced below or raised above the normal—which proceeding must decidedly and enduringly influence the internal temperature of the body—we have the direct retarding or enhancing influence referred to.

"That an increased consumption of oxygen is a manifestation of the application of cold has been clearly shown by Rohrig and Zuntz.

. . . .

"My clinical observation in the Montefiore Home, which receives only incurable cases, confirms the views of Winternitz, that an improvement in the general condition and weight of a large number of cases whose hoplessness has been attested by previous unsuccessful treatment and by every diagnostic sign, is proof that cold water applications, carefully adapted to each case, improve the appetite, deepen the respiration, refresh every organ, and thus infuse an increased energy into the glandular and other functions which contribute to tissue metamorphosis."

Thus it is proved that the bath not only cleanses and, as we say, stimulates the skin, but it exercises a direct influence upon the entire system, increasing its activity and encouraging the combustion of used up material and its removal from the body. Every one recognizes the necessity of bathing the face and hands at least once a day. It is just as important for the rest of the body.

If impracticable to bathe the entire body

every morning, at least bathe face, neck, chest, and back, to aid in preventing secretions which might cause catarrhal or tubercular deposit from remaining near the respiratory organs. It is also obviously necessary that the groins be bathed night and morning.

The temperature of the apartment where the bath is taken should be from sixty-four to seventy-four degrees Fahrenheit, and the water fully as cold, in early days of cold bathing, and should be reduced to a much lower temperature when the skin has become disciplined to the change from the warmer bath.

The hand is an excellent wash-cloth, and should always be employed for the face and neck. Loosely woven material of silk or wool is preferable to cotton. A sponge should never be used, especially in bathing the eyes and ears, or any open sores; not only for the reason that the texture is harsh and unsympathetic in touch, but because impurities lodge in the recesses, and it can only be safely used after it has been plunged in disinfectants. A rotary motion is better than the common method of rubbing, both to stimulate the pores of the skin and the capillary circulation. Dry the skin quickly by using a soft towel. Do not redden it by rough friction, as the pores are thus irritated, and their functions thereby interrupted. The "glow" some persons enjoy is not healthful for the skin, if produced by the friction of a harsh towel. More cuticle is removed than is easily rebuilt, although some phenomenal cases exist where the velvety texture has not been destroyed by this treatment. It is desirable that a certain amount of cuticle be removed daily, but the rotation with the hand gives this result without irritating the pores, as does the rough treatment referred to.

The flesh-brush, except for hands and feet, is injurious for daily bathing. Its safe use is only in the Turkish bath, where subsequent massage obviates irritation that would otherwise ensue.

The daily use of soap, except where it is obviously necessary, is unwise, as it dries out too much of the oleaginous element of the skin, causing greater demands on the nutrient arteries in replacing the loss, and the other tissues are in consequence imperfectly supplied. Besides, unless thoroughly washed off, it leaves another kind of dirt in the pores. One complete soap bath a week is sufficient for the daily bather.

Warm baths sap the system too heavily. They also render the skin devoid of tone, and the pores of contractility. If the warm bath is at any time indulged in, it should be followed by a cold shower or rapid cold sponge.

Tri-daily baths are harmful, as the skin cannot rebuild fast enough to counteract the destruction of cuticle thus occasioned.

I will suggest a simple basin bath, safe for the delicate, and, if facilities are lacking for more complete bathing, sufficient for the more robust.

This entire bath occupies only from five to ten minutes, as a thorough wetting and drying are all that is necessary, except on mornings of the soap bath.

It is best for women to wear vest and gown at night, and, whenever leaving the bed, to step into woollen slippers, else chills are apt to result from the sensitive sole of the foot coming in contact with the cold floor. This is especially necessary with the delicate.

Weak tissues should receive the first dash of cold water. The shock is a splendid nerve stimulant, and also localizes the blood current. Begin, then, the basin bath as follows:

Wash and dry the face, employing the rotary motion previously referred to. The bath for neck and ears comes next. Then remove the arms from the gown, and tie it by the sleeves around the waist.

Wash and dry the arms.

Remove the vest, wash and dry the chest, shoulders, and the body to the waist.

Replace the gown to prevent chilling, and finish the bath under the gown, bathing and drying the lower body, then the thighs, and then the legs and feet.

By this process the circulation is carried evenly downward, the skin is sufficiently cleansed, and no harm can result. Dressing should immediately follow, and the individual is then in readiness for the morning meal.

Providing this proves too fatiguing for a very delicate person, she would better fortify herself by drinking some nourishing beverage, as bovox or warm milk, before arising; or, perhaps, take but a partial bath (face, neck, and chest) before breakfast, finishing the rest an hour or two afterward. In any and every case discontinue the custom of night bathing except feet, groins, and arm-pits for cleanliness, especially with children. Make all changes gradually, not radically, lest they prove more detrimental than beneficial to health.

The cold foot bath in hot weather is sometimes very refreshing at night, and induces sleep.

For baby's bath see chapter on Early Life and Training of Children.

Turkish baths are a luxury all should take occasion to enjoy. They should be taken with discretion, however, and the physician in charge ought to understand the heart action of each patron, adjusting treatment accordingly. They are, we must remember, of therapeutic advantage to the thin rather than the stout. The treatment, of course, accelerates combustion, but it also encourages tissue growth.

Oil baths are excellent for the emaciated or poorly nourished, but it must be borne in mind that good massage should accompany them, or the pores will be obstructed rather than nourished.

Air baths, *i. e.*, massage in a current of fresh air (warmed, if necessary), are also valuable remedial agents.

Alcohol baths should be very judiciously taken, else too great destruction of tissue results, and too much of the nutritive element is consumed.

Sea baths, if not positively harmful, are generally beneficial. The salt water has a healthful action on the skin, and the shock of the cold plunge is health-giving, if one is in condition to endure it. It should be remembered that the exercise of surf bathing is exceedingly violent, and care should be taken that it is not overdone. In this, rather than the chill, lies the greatest danger.

There is a great temptation, however, to remain too long in the water, and most persons regulate the length of their bath by their comfort, leaving only when they feel cold. This is very wrong. A bath of fifteen minutes' duration is enough for any ordinary person, even in quiet weather, and when the water is rough it should be much shortened. Weak or delicate persons should seldom take more than a few plunges and come out at once. Care should be taken to select a good, dry, airy bath-house. Generally, beaches are deficient in this respect.

CHAPTER XXVIII

CARE OF THE COMPLEXION

"I long not for the cherries on the tree
So much as those which on a lip I see;
And more affection bear I to the rose
That in a cheek than in a garden grows."
—RANDOLPH.

A PERFECT woman nobly planned, with health and beauty well preserved, is the best ornament of the home. It is, therefore, not only her right, but also her duty, to see that her personal attractiveness does not wane with the progress of time.

Health and beauty go hand in hand together. Without health there is seldom any enduring beauty; yet it is a mistake to suppose that mere rude health is an all-sufficient beautifier, and, possessing that, to suffer facial lines to form and deepen, and the tiny pores to enlarge until the whole fine texture of the skin is coarsened. These are grim traces which time leaves when allowed to approach as a destroyer.

No skill in tasteful costuming can successfully conceal or counteract the impression produced by these ravages.

Nowadays the rational woman and the thoughtful girl are alike desirous of knowing what unfavorable influences to avoid, what practices to abolish, and what hygienic measures to adopt, in order to restore or preserve firmness and shapeliness of muscles, smoothness of outline, and velvety texture of skin. In this chapter I shall aim to cover these points.

The causes to which defects in the complexion are traceable are as numerous as those leading to defective health, and study of the individual is necessary in order to accurately prescribe treatment. If proper conditions of health are attained, and the facial tissues do not respond to the general treatment here recommended and take on their natural beauty, then the advice of an able specialist had best be sought.

The practice of what are erroneously styled "facial gymnastics" is a deadly enemy to comeliness. They create and accentuate disfiguring lines in both face and throat. Lines form when the connective tissue which attaches muscle to bone becomes over-strengthened or hardened, forming a groove into which the skin shapes itself. Instead, therefore, of practicing exercises that contract these muscles the more, it is necessary to employ a method for softening and normalizing the connective tissue by means of enforced circulation. Head movements, massage, and passive work are the only desirable exercises for improving the face muscles. They may be performed either by the patient herself, or by an attendant.

The use of such devices as irritating washes, plasters, masks, and poultices is another baneful practice. The theory upon which these and the bleaching compounds are advertised and put forth is, that irritants remove the impaired cuticle, and that a fresh and youthful skin will grow to replace the former disfigured one. But whether the wash, mixture, or appliance is composed of chemical ingredients, or merely contains lemon juice, alcohol, or alkali, remember that in the economy of nature more tissue should not be removed than can be easily and quickly rebuilt; and the punishment of a worn-out skin will sooner or later follow this harmful practice. Of course some phenomenal exceptions prove this rule in error;

but the advice given here is not for the exceptions, but for the majority, to whom it cannot fail to be of service.

Internal remedies are even more pernicious than those for external application. Drugs should not be taken into the system, save on the recommendation of competent medical authority. Amateur advice and advertised skin treatment should alike be submitted to the family physician for approval.

The fear of age is a potent destroyer of beauty. A morbid consciousness of growing old, and dread and worriment because of it, add more and deeper lines than the actual advance of time. A woman is the age she appears to be, to paraphrase the old saying, and the woman of fifty, healthy and beautiful in mind and body, is at once more interesting to, and more admired by, her friends of both sexes, than the woman of half her years who is a pessimistic semi-invalid, with views and values of life as disordered as her internal economy, and as unlovely as her neglected face.

Some speak of youth as though all of a woman's charm must fade and fail as it passes away. But if youthfulness is the only foundation for her claim to attractiveness, it is certain that she can at no period appeal to any beyond a very inferior circle.

Men frequently amuse themselves by tales of women denying their age, and setting back the scale of birthday progression. Women themselves have given impetus to this form of ridicule by making their birthdays but milestones to decay and degeneracy. The jealous woman often watches and points out how other women's beauty fades, not realizing that the men whom she thus seeks to prejudice will thereby learn to discern the same signs in herself.

Facial lines are deepened every time the expression by which they were originally traced, flits over the countenance. As already explained, the connective tissue attaching muscle to bone becomes over-strengthened by much exercise in any direction, and therefore the habitual expressions write their character most strongly upon the face. It is unfortunately the fact that such records do not indicate a predominance of happiness, contentment, peace. Let the woman who would be beautiful remember always that her thoughts rather than her cosmetics or her clothes decide her facial attractiveness. Then, instead of fear, dread, anxiety, anger, scorn, ill-temper, jealousy, cynicism, and other painful and trying emotions, hope, courage, faith, and good cheer will inscribe bright legends, whose winsomeness is safe from the withering touch of time.

A careful perusal of the preceding chapters will impart valuable instruction concerning the preservation of the skin texture. Consider first the influence of good digestion. It is indisputable that sour stomachs produce sour looks, to say nothing of the influence on skin texture. Living in ill-ventilated rooms has a bad effect on the skin; and thin-soled shoes and insufficient clothing, which admit of chilliness from damp or cold, cause contraction of the muscles, with consequent deepening of wrinkles, marking of lines, and enlarging and coarsening of pores, till the condition we designate as "goose-flesh," is established.

Neither drugs nor cosmetics can remedy such wrongs once visited upon the skin. The only hope rests in normalizing the texture by rational hygienic means, and then preserving it by proper care.

Under ordinary conditions, the face needs washing but once a day, and that in the morning. Use a silk or wool wash-cloth in preference to cotton or sponge; but the palmar surfaces of the hands are preferable to either. Manipulation during the bath is invaluable. Employ the rotary movement, described in the chapter on Massage, and spend fully five minutes on the face bath. Plenty of rotation on the lines will go far toward obliterating them.

It is not generally known that the prone position usually assumed when one stoops over the basin to bathe the face is bad for the muscles. Massage should not be given to sagging muscles; instead, they should be distended, to avoid congestion. Hold the face erect during the manipulation, that the blood may circulate properly. This posture will also accelerate the passage of venous blood, which would be retarded were the muscles in a lax or sagging condition.

The face should be dried with a soft towel, applied with a rotary motion. Do not drag the muscles downward in the process.

For the "oily skin" of which many complain, frequent manipulation with dry fingers will almost certainly prove advantageous. It helps to normalize open pores, restores the functions of weak sebaceous glands, and by improving the capillary circulation aids in rebuilding the tissues. The movement should be upward and outward, moving the skin on the muscles, not rubbing upon the surface of the skin.

A paste of fine table salt moistened with water or milk, is a valuable stimulant for a healthy skin, but should not be used if any disease is present. This should not be applied oftener than once a week. Rub it well over the face. Then wash it off thoroughly, and dry with a soft towel. This sand-papers off some of the cuticle, and, by stimulating the papillæ and capillary circulation, promotes healthy growth.

I will now outline a simple formula of face massage which, followed at night, will be especially beneficial, as the night's repose is a valuable aid in tissue building. It also brings a sense of restfulness to the tired mind, by directing the thoughts to the treatment, and thereby withdrawing them from other subjects, possibly vexatious ones; and the circulation thus stimulated relieves the overcharged blood-vessels of the brain, by drawing the current to the surface.

If practiced before going out in a dry, strong

wind, it will tend to preserve the texture of the skin from chapping; and repeating it on returning indoors will normalize its condition. A cream made of vegetable oils, combined with some simple astringent, should be used. It will cleanse and nourish the pores, and prevent any irritation that might attend the vigorous massage.

PRESCRIPTION I. FOR FACE MASSAGE.

1. Apply light touches of cream on the face, and rotate it thoroughly into the pores of the skin.

2. Direct the movement from the centre of the forehead upward and outward each way; from under the eyes work lightly outward toward the temples. The tissues here are extremely delicate, and must not be fingered as roughly as the cheeks, forehead, and chin.

3. Rotate much at the base of the nose, and over the nostrils. The skin here is apt to coarsen, and the pores enlarge to the size of pin-holes, making a very ugly appearance, which this treatment is pretty certain to modify, if not entirely remove.

4. After rotating the whole surface of the

face and neck with the fingers, as directed, stroke heavily, using the palmar surface of the four fingers of both hands at once, making the passes from the centre of the forehead outward, and back of the ears downward on the veins at the side of the neck; also upward at the sides of the mouth and nose, and from the chin to the ears, to empty the veins, and promote better circulation. (See chart of head veins, chapter XXII., Massage.) Dry off the cream that remains on the surface, by rotating with a soft towel. Then rotate a few moments with dry fingers, and stroke softly.

This process should occupy from twenty to thirty minutes, if faithfully followed; but even a five-minute treatment, when no more time can be spared, will be of substantial benefit. It will leave the skin peculiarly soft and velvety, a condition which in a little while becomes permanent.

Dr. Benjamin Lee speaks especially of the efficacy of massage in restoring a dry, harsh skin to a condition of softness, pliability, and healthy moisture. He also speaks of its wonderful advantage in skin diseases, and quotes Shoemaker as authority. It is a science that certainly invites research, one that should not be tabooed merely because it has suffered from inferior labor, or because some obstinate cases of disease did not yield to its application.

PRESCRIPTION II.

In connection with the foregoing prescription, about once a week, after giving the massage recommended, the face should be bathed with hot water and soap, then dashed with cold water, and dried in the manner already described. Rotate a little with the fingers, and if the washing has left the skin too dry, use a touch of cream, applied as aforesaid.

This process is wonderfully beautifying, and is recommended for occasions when a woman wishes to appear especially at her best, but should not be repeated oftener than twice a week.

In place of prescription II., face steaming may be resorted to; but it is not safe to practice it unless one has been properly instructed. The time of the steaming should not exceed five minutes, and three minutes generally suffices for delicate skins. This question, however, is determined by the texture of the skin, the reactive power and the health of the individual. Thorough massage must follow the steaming. Without it nothing but harm can result. Properly administered, steaming rejuvenates the complexion, and so softens the muscles that better results are obtained from the after massage. Without rational care, it removes too much of the natural juices of the skin, and eventually renders the tissues dry and lifeless. It is only in rare and exceptional cases that face-steaming should be given more frequently than once a week.

If the processes above described fail to remove "blackheads," it is best to obtain more specific advice.

Those desiring to reduce superfluous adipose of chin—double-chin, as it is commonly called—must rotate the muscles heavily, stroking in the direction of the large veins (see plate XCI.).

Those who seek to build up lacking tissues, and to fill out hollows, will have to manipulate with lighter, more persuasive touches, and frequently.

The treatment described is effective in modifying the wrinkled, drooping condition of the skin, and to a certain extent the deep sharp wrinkles as well; but a specific manipulation will secure more speedy results for these. It is as follows:

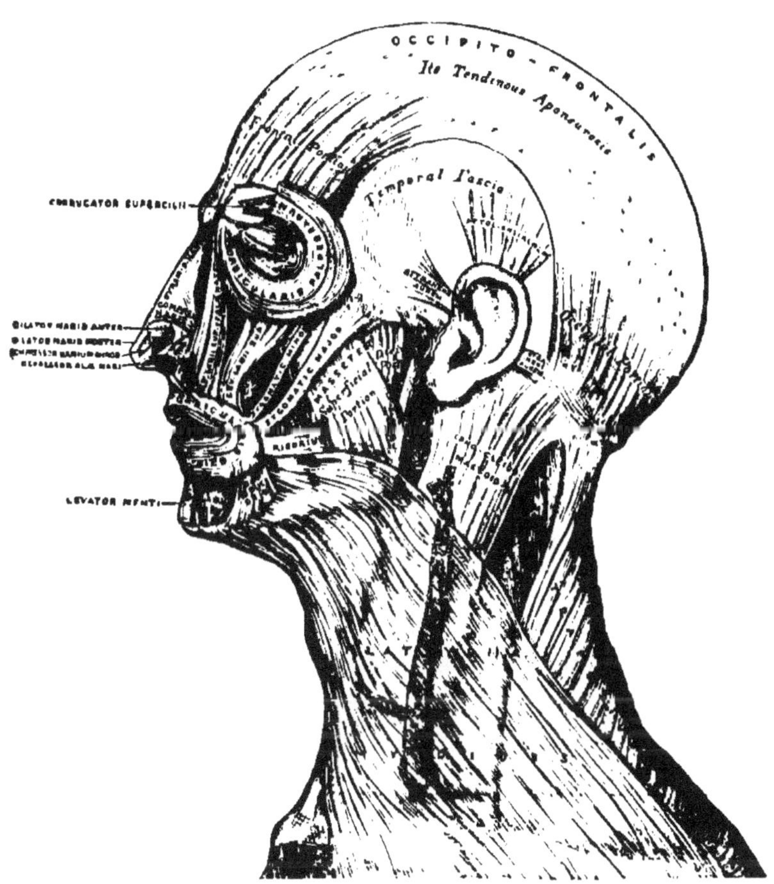
OCCIPITO - FRONTALIS
Its Tendinous Aponeurosis
Temporal Fascia
CORRUGATOR SUPERCILII
LEVATOR MENTI

XCVIII.

PRESCRIPTION III.

1. With the palmar surface of either the first, second, or third fingers, whichever is most convenient, rub with a cross stroke into the groove, the fingers held side by side, but moving in opposite directions.

2. For the lines that in later years are apt to extend from the base of the ear, down the throat, begin at the lowest point, and with this movement rub upward to the ear, pressing well into the deep line to render flexible the stiff muscle and the connective tissue. Bear in mind that the treatment is to soften and normalize these tissues.

These throat lines are not necessarily age-marks, but are often due to a wrong carriage of the head. "Poking the chin," and holding the head too rigidly will cause them, by putting an undue strain upon the side throat muscles. This posture of the head also causes baggy cheeks. The exercises prescribed under the "head movements" are adapted to counteract these tendencies.

3. The horizontal wrinkles upon the forehead should be treated with the same cross stroke, directing the movement from the centre out-

ward to the temples. Perpendicular lines, as between the eyes, should be worked upwards. Pressure is required in this line treatment.

4. For minute lines or wrinkles under the eyes, the cross stroke should be used, but the fingers must be held diagonally, to guard against pressure upon the eyeball. The touch should be light and even.

A home massage machine which I have invented, and shall patent, gives all the movements described, and spares the physical exertion of using the hands. This appliance is easily portable, may be operated from any ordinary table, and has attachments adapted for use upon all parts of the body, as well as upon the face and neck.

To return to the subject of the face bath. Soft water should invariably be used for bathing. A small quantity of borax, a bag of wheat bran, or one of almond meal, will help to soften it.

Use whatever soap agrees best with the individual skin, providing it is pure and not scented. Scented soaps are not as apt to be pure as are the unscented. Almond meal often takes the place of soap in the bath.

The selection of toilet creams involves careful

study. Those containing vaseline and glycerine are best avoided, for the reason that these properties are very apt to promote hair-growth on the face. Lead and other chemicals are even more harmful. Vegetable oils, with simple astringents, are the requisites for the manufacture of face creams. What the skin needs most is care. It will not thrive if the pores are dried with soap, clogged by creams, or obstructed by powders.

The use of electricity for the complexion is favorable or pernicious according to the condition of the patient and the ability of the electrician. The faradic current does not improve the skin, and the stimulation is apt to deepen the lines. I know of many instances where this has been the result. The galvanic current is beneficial in many cases, but should never be tolerated, except at the hands of a person skilled in therapeutics, as well as in the technique of electricity. The art of electro-facial massage is as yet chiefly in the hands of the unskilled, who have chosen this practice because they are in need of some means of livelihood, not from possessing any especial adaptability to the art. It is a great risk to submit one's self to the treatment of these untrained operators, whose methods are crude experiments rather than the result of wise experience, or even of intelligent experiment. Better study Nature's laws for yourself, and obey them, and not allow electrical and other quacks to operate on your complexion to the probable injury and possible destruction of whatever beauty belongs to it.

CHAPTER XXIX

CARE OF THE HAIR

"A woman's hair is her crown of glory."

GRAVE injuries to the general health, and detriment to the preservation of the hair are consequent upon indiscriminate head baths. The skin of the head, like that of the body, requires daily treatment, to keep the pores in good working order and to stimulate the capillary circulation; but unlike the skin of the body, it is not benefited by daily bathing. We must, therefore, seek advantage through massage. The manipulation for the scalp comprises a vigorous rotary movement, performed with the palmar surfaces of the fingers of both hands, followed by a downward stroking to empty the veins, if the treatment has called too much blood to the head. Begin the movement at the top of the head, and direct it downward to the base of the brain; also from the temples backward and downward. If there is tendency to congestive headaches, much vigorous massage should be given at the base of the brain, followed by crosswise rubbing on the back of the neck. (See chapter on Massage.)

Substitute for this, at discretion, vigorous treatment with a hair brush. Select a brush with bristles of average length and stiffness. Part the hair at intervals, and rub the scalp thoroughly with the brush. After sufficiently stimulating the scalp in this way, brush the hair with long, careful strokes, to remove the dust. The scalp, rather than the hair, should receive the greater amount of attention.

Either the brushing or the massage should be an established daily custom. Even five minutes will be of great benefit, if no more time can be allowed for it. It stimulates the activity of the glands, removes impurities thrown off through the pores, and obviates the necessity for frequent washing. Dr. E. W. Brooke of Philadelphia says of this treatment: "It promotes hair growth, excites the action of the hair cells, and prevents absorption of the fatty and muscular layers forming the scalp, arrests atrophy of the hair bulbs, and, by increasing the circulation, prevents the hair from turning gray." We are indebted to her for substantiated theories which place a therapeutic and hygienic value on scalp massage equal to that which Dr. Lee attributes to general massage.

To free the hair from tangles, begin at the head and work downward. The ends will be less split and worn if unnecessary combing is spared.

Leave the hair loose at night, especially if confined during the day. A silk handkerchief worn loosely over the head at night imparts gloss to the hair, and affords protection from draught to people of neuralgic tendency, besides helping generate electricity.

In case the hair is falling, moisten the scalp with touches of an oil made of three parts vaseline to one part lanoline, well mixed; rotate it thoroughly into the pores of the skin. Do this for half an hour, or more, at night, and repeat the rubbing next morning without applying any more vaseline. This treatment once a week is sure to do good, and in most cases will prove, with the daily massage, a sufficient check to the loss of hair, and will also prevent its turning gray.

Well-regulated toilet-tables now boast a small instrument of the brush variety, not larger than a paint brush. It is for applying vaseline to the eyebrows. Vaseline is reputed to be an excellent ointment for making both eyebrows and eyelashes grow.

The hair should be clipped several times each year, to remove split ends and help promote the growth. A convenient way to do this is as follows:

Braid the hair loosely in two or more braids, and draw these "the wrong way" through the hand, to loosen out the ends of uneven hair along the whole length, and clip the loosened ends.

This should be done often or seldom, according to the growth and condition of hair. That of a slow, firm growth will not require it more than once in six months; while that of more rapid growth, or the hair prone to split ends, will require it every month. "The new moon" is a good traditional date, and allows about the right interval.

Sufficient attention to heavy hair requires much time and strength, and the services of a maid is really needful. If, however, such aid is impossible, it is best to lessen the quantity of hair, cutting off and out the excess in length and weight, and keeping only what is necessary for a becoming *coiffure*.

With the above directions followed daily, head baths are not a frequent necessity. Intervals of from two to three months may elapse between them. Too frequent head baths exhaust the nutrient elements of the sebaceous glands, and in time the hair growth fails from imperfect nourishment. Particularly should dry hair be spared from frequent washing. The oily scalp should be washed more frequently, but even this condition is greatly benefited by the massage. No woman can afford to lose this crown of beauty for which there is no satisfactory substitute. Artificial compromises are always apparent.

Hygienic rules should be carefully observed in the head bath, especially in the drying process, as many neuralgic and congestive headaches, besides colds, causing exaggeration of inherent ills, result from lack of proper attention to them.

In the head bath, first wet thoroughly the hair and scalp. Soap is not necessary, but, if any is to be used, white castile is preferred; it should be dissolved in hot water, and the hair, as well as the scalp, thoroughly rubbed with the solution.

An egg, both yolk and white, beaten with

about two tablespoonfuls of water, rubbed into the scalp, strengthens the hair growth, removes dandruff, and hardens the scalp. The yolk of the egg is a tonic, and supplies iron and sulphur; and the white is an alkali, which, combined with the oil of the hair, makes sufficient soap for cleansing it. Rub this well into the scalp. Some specialists prefer having the yolk and white rubbed in singly, the yolk first, followed by thorough treatment with the white.

After either application, rinse with warm water, and, when the cleansing is completed, gradually reduce the temperature of the water until it is quite cold. This will prevent taking cold in the head.

The towel shampoo follows. When this is thoroughly done, the hair is ready for complete and easy drying. It should be shaken in little strands, and tossed about over the shoulders until thoroughly dry. Alternate this treatment with frequent scalp rotation, to stimulate capillary circulation.

The process here described is safe for even the most delicate, but it must be continued until the hair, especially at the base of the brain, is perfectly dry.

Artificial heat is injurious, as it not only

draws too much blood to the head, and makes the hair brittle, but renders the tissues susceptible to colds.

Fanning the hair cannot be generally recommended. It is apt to bring on colds and neuralgia. The woman who cannot take time for rational attention to her head bath would better rely entirely on the daily manipulation. A small quantity of vaseline and lanoline should be rotated into the scalp after the drying process is complete, to supply what oil has been removed by the bath.

Too great caution in the care of the hair cannot be exercised. Let me emphasize my previous remark that many neuralgic and congestive headaches, besides colds, causing exaggeration of other ills, follow indiscriminate head baths. Many cases are on record of health being wrecked through a girl's washing her hair when her physical conditions were unfavorable.

CHAPTER XXX

EMERGENCY WORK, AND FIRST AID TO THE INJURED

"But a certain Samaritan, as he journeyed, came where he was: and when he saw him, he had compassion on him, and went to him and bound up his wounds."—LUKE X. 33, 34.

IN every walk of life, especially in every school and home, there is the crying need of instruction in emergency work. There are no limitations to the accidents that may at any time occur, and that demand from us proper and immediate care. Sprained ankles, severe bruises from falls, cuts, bites, cases of fainting, drowning, epileptic fits, poisoning, etc., are daily brought to our notice, to say nothing of disastrous railroad accidents where scores of human beings are seriously maimed, and where the services of the amateur educated in general knowledge of "what to do while awaiting the arrival of the physician or surgeon" are invaluable. A few minutes' profuse arterial bleeding may deplete the system beyond years of recuperation, or even cause loss of a life, while timely aid would have saved it. A sprained ankle properly masséed and bandaged by the amateur, at the time of the accident, may regain strength in a few days, while as many months would not otherwise restore it. Everybody, especially mothers and teachers, should be educated to dress a simple wound and attend to shock, and, in severe cases, to at least keep the patient in good condition of mind and body until able services can be obtained. Instead of this, it is a deplorable fact that most women and girls either faint at sight of blood, or stand helplessly around, adding distress to the scene by whispered remarks and sad faces, influences that have an exceedingly depressing effect on the patient, and are, to say the least, unwomanly. Is it right that the girls are graduated as finished women of a great nation, when the sight of blood causes them to faint, and when, with their hands educated in every other fine art, they are powerless to render efficient aid in disaster?

Dr. Glentworth R. Butler, of Brooklyn, N.Y., has written a practical, concise handbook, entitled " Emergency Notes; What to do in Accident and Sudden Illness until the Doctor Comes." The title alone recommends it, and it should certainly be in the possession of every mother and teacher in the land. He was my first instructor in this valuable work.

In this chapter I have space to make but a few suggestions, which I hope will lead the reader to study the subject more thoroughly. This chapter is an outline of subjects for study rather than a study of any of the subjects.

I will first describe the use of the triangular bandage, which is the most practical in the hands of the amateur. It is made of a piece of light-weight muslin (unbleached is best for the purpose) eighteen to thirty-six inches square, according to size of part to be bandaged, cut diagonally across, making two triangles of the square. The handkerchief folded serves the same purpose, and the school child should be taught its use. It may be used as a triangle for holding a hand, foot, or chest application; as a cravat, *i. e.*, folded with apex against the diagonal base, and two or three more folds to give the shape its name indicates; as an arm sling; or as a cord for improvised tourniquet. (See cuts XCIX. and C.) If you wish to go farther into the subject, the roller bandage offers a field for quite extensive study.

Bandages may be fastened with stitches, pins, or knots. Stitches are best, and knots

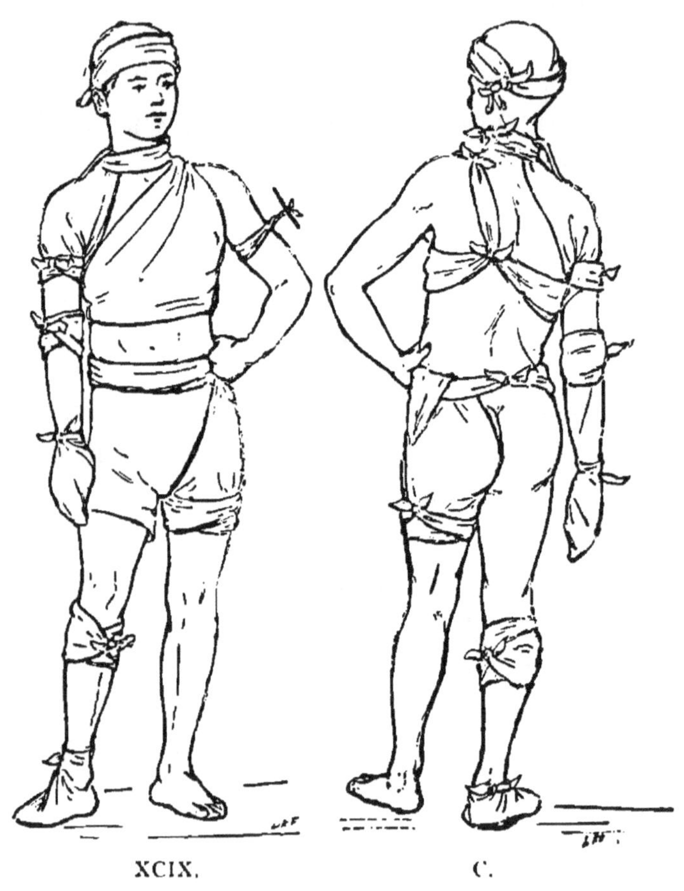

XCIX. C.

are least desirable. If knots are used, take care that they do not press against any large blood-vessels or nerve trunks, or on sensitive tissues, and that the smooth side is against the patient. A bandage should be firm, but not tight.

The first care for the injured is to stop bleeding (in case of open wound), attend to shock, and send quickly for the physician. Retain a few willing, practical assistants, but allow no curious or sad-faced lookers-on. Maintain calm presence of mind, give the patient courage, and avoid expressing sympathy.

We designate wounds as follows: *lacerated*, when caused by a bruising or tearing instrument, as from machine or railroad injury, or a bite; *incised*, when a cut is made with a sharp cutting instrument. A *contusion* is when the injury is under the skin.

Press the fingers into a lacerated wound, to stop profuse bleeding. Press one finger above and one below an incised wound, pressing the edges together, and bandage tightly. In either case, ice, very cold water, or hot water—one hundred and fifteen to one hundred and twenty-five degrees—will aid in checking the bleeding. Avoid lukewarm water. It will cause the blood to flow more freely. Elevating the injured member also aids by gravitation in retarding the bleeding. If these measures are not satisfactory, apply the improvised tourniquet; *i. e.*, tie a handkerchief loosely around the wounded member, between the injury and the heart, and twist tightly with a pencil or stick, to stop the blood current that supplies the wound. Fasten one end of the stick under the tourniquet, to hold it in position while the wound is being bandaged. In severe cases, leave the tourniquet adjusted until the physician arrives. Avoid astringents such as iron, alum, or tannin, and especially such clogging substances as cobwebs. At best they can only check capillary bleeding, which is never serious, and they greatly interfere with the healing of a wound.

If foreign matter has lodged in a wound, as is generally the case, cleanse it carefully before dressing it. If there has been severe bleeding which has stopped, do not wash away clotted blood; the physician will attend to that. (See chapter on Circulation.) The clot is nature's method of stopping a ruptured blood-vessel, and is often a successful one, even in severe cases of bleeding. The arteries, in addition to the other characteristics above described, have a most remarkable faculty which operates with the clot and serves to keep it in place. When an artery is severed, the edges, at the place where the cut occurs, contract toward each other, and thus make the opening smaller. The clot forms immediately inside this contracted opening, and the edges so folded inward hold it in place and prevent its being forced out, except by considerable pressure. Hence the necessity of encouraging clotting, and of preventing sudden or violent jars or jolts, or anything which forces the blood more rapidly, such as exertion or excitement.

Use a clean cloth (a handkerchief, fresh from the laundry) in washing a wound. Never use a sponge. Impurities are apt to be retained in its meshes, and to cause pus formation in the wound. Vinegar and water (one part vinegar to four parts water), carbolic acid (one teaspoonful to a teacup of water), or common salt, same proportion, will be a valuable antiseptic to use in cleansing a wound.

If the head is injured, cut the hair close with the first touch of the scissors; do not chop it by degrees, as the hair particles are hard to remove.

In closing a wound with plaster, use strips,

so that the wound may discharge. Absorbent cotton or a muslin pad, wet with some of the above mentioned solutions, extract of witch hazel and water, or listerine, should be placed on the wound before adjusting the bandage.

A sprained ankle had best be submerged in water as hot as can be borne, or bound with ice for a full half hour; stroke, meanwhile, up the legs, to empty the veins and induce capillary circulation, and thereby prevent congestion. (See chapter on Massage.) Bandage tightly, and at intervals remove the bandage; repeat the treatment and bandage again. Skilled massage is better than the hot water or ice treatment. The amateur can give much relief, by rotating the skin on the muscle around (perhaps not on) the injury, and stroking upward to empty the veins.

A fractured bone or dislocated joint had best not be disturbed by the amateur. There is great danger of causing the splintered end of the bone to pierce the flesh, causing a compound fracture, which is more difficult to treat. Cut away the clothing, and make the patient comfortable. If necessary to move the patient, prop the injured member with soft pillows; improvise a splint of any convenient article, a book, folded newspaper, piece of a box, or umbrella well padded, and fastened on with the handkerchief bandage. For this it is best to cut the bandage material straightwise, in inch wide strips, from each side to within three inches of centre; place this under the splint, and tie the opposite ends firmly around; a small pillow or cushion folded around the fractured member, and fastened with this, or with triangular bandages, will serve the amateur well in caring for an injury of this description.

Dislocations are not as easily made comfortable. It is best not to put on bandage or splint unless it is absolutely necessary for transporting the patient.

Shock, to a greater or less degree, usually attends injury. In some cases it is very slight, and no special attention is necessary. In others it is a dangerous condition. The symptoms are pallor, clamminess, and loss of consciousness. Hot applications to feet, arm-pits, and pit of stomach are needed. Stimulants in very moderate quantities may be given. Brandy (a teaspoonful to a half cup of hot water), or aromatic spirits of ammonia (ten drops to a half cup of hot water), given at intervals of ten to twenty minutes, are all the amateur should attempt.

Stimulants must never be given when there are open, bleeding wounds. The reason is obvious. They accelerate the bleeding.

For burns and scalds, apply a saturated solution or paste of baking soda, or olive oil, lard, vaseline, or equal parts raw linseed oil and lime water. The object is to prevent air from reaching the burned surface.

I will quote, by permission, from Dr. Butler's book on treatment for resuscitation in cases of suspended animation, also for poisoning and poisonous bites.

DROWNING.

"Immersion even for one minute has destroyed life. On the other hand, pearl and sponge divers remain under water for two or three minutes, having acquired such ability by continued practice.

"There are two kinds of cases met with. In the first, as soon as the person falls into the water, a condition which resembles fainting ensues. The heart beats very feebly. The breathing stops, and no water is drawn into the air passages. Restoration to life is more probable than in the second kind, where fainting does not occur, and in an attempt to breathe while immersed, water is drawn into the windpipe and lungs.

"There are certain things which are of great importance to remember if any one is in danger of drowning, always provided that he can retain self-control and presence of mind. The body, as a whole, is lighter than water, and will float if the arms and greater part of the head remain under water. Therefore, if any one is in this danger, he should lie flat on the back, keep the arms under water, stretched full length above the head, expire and inspire quickly, holding the air in the lungs after inspiration as long as possible, so as to keep them filled during the greater part of the time.

Then wait quietly for assistance. Struggling and throwing the arms out of water will cause the person to sink.

RULES FOR THE TREATMENT OF THE APPARENTLY DROWNED.

"Never stop working until a physician pronounces the case hopeless.

"Remember that the patient is suffering from two things—want of air or oxygen, and loss of heat from the body. Want of oxygen is the pressing need which must be supplied; therefore, if the patient is not breathing, artificial respiration should be commenced and continued, first, last, and all the time. Begin and carry on your work in the following order:

"1. Cut and tear the clothing from the upper part of the body, to give freedom of movement.

"2. Keep in the open air, if the weather permits.

"3. Turn the body on the face, forehead resting on hand, to keep mouth clear of ground. Place a coat or two, made into a roll, under stomach and hips, in order to have a sloping line from base of lungs to mouth. In absence of roll, stand astride of patient, grasp hips and raise high. This will allow water to run out of the windpipe. Assist it by placing a hand on each side of spine, at back of chest, and pressing forcibly two or three times. Let this occupy not more than one minute.

"4. Turn body on the back. Place roll of clothing under the shoulders. The roll may be dispensed with, if not procurable.

"5. Wrap handkerchief around forefinger, pass into the mouth and clean out mucus. Grasp tip of tongue and draw it forward and down on chin. Have some one hold it there; or, if alone, lay a strip of material on tongue, pass the ends behind the neck, and tie. Otherwise the tongue may fall back and close the throat.

"6. Then begin artificial respiration (Sylvester's method). Kneel at patient's head.

"*First Movement* (*Inspiration*).—Grasp arms at or just below the elbows. Bring the arms

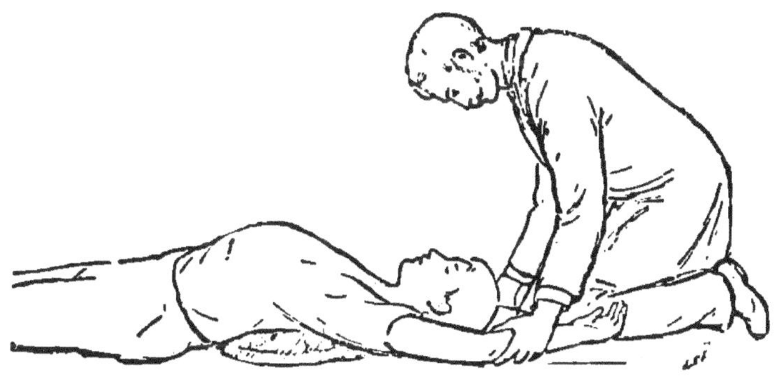

CI.

up over head and down to the ground, so that the elbows touch the ground. Hold them there for three seconds, or while you count one, two, three, rather slowly. The muscles attached to the upper arm-bone and to the ribs pull upon the latter so as to expand the chest, and air enters the lungs. (See CI.)

" *Second Movement* (*Expiration*).—From this position carry arms down so that the elbows rest one upon either side of the front of the chest. Let the weight of your body bear upon

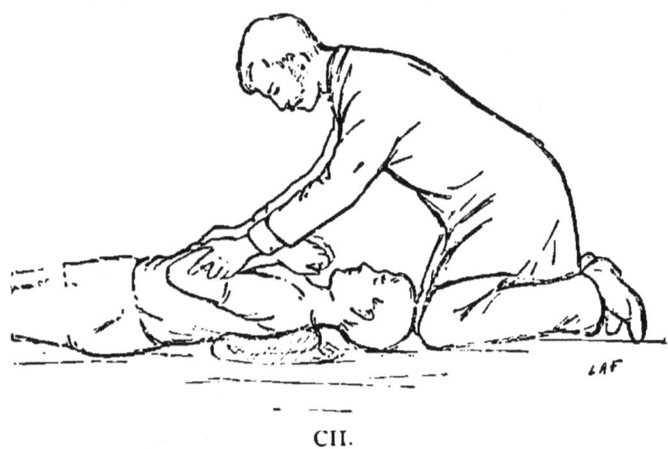

CII.

the chest and ribs, while you count one, two, three, rather slowly, as if you were endeavoring to squeeze the air out of the lungs, which is, in fact, precisely what you wish to do. (See CII.)

" The preceding points are most important.

But the patient is also suffering from loss of heat; therefore, if you have others to aid you,

"7. Send for warmed blankets and quilts, bottles or rubber bags filled with hot water; for bricks, stones, bags of sand or salt heated in the oven.

"8. Send also for brandy, whiskey, wine, or aromatic spirits of ammonia, to be used when patient can swallow.

"9. While you are continuing artificial respiration, let others remove the remaining wet clothing, apply heat by methods referred to, and rub the limbs vigorously upward.

"10. From time to time stop artificial respiration for a moment, in order to see whether the patient is himself attempting to breathe. Change of color in the face, gasping, or movement of the pit of the stomach, are favorable signs. If he begins to breathe, do not hinder him by squeezing air out of the lungs when he is making an effort to get it in. Slap the bare chest with a towel wet in cold water, or, better, pour hot and cold water alternately on the chest. Either of these will stimulate the breathing, as any one who has gasped under a cold shower bath will testify. In addition, apply smelling-salts or ammonia to the nostrils.

"11. As soon as the patient can swallow, give stimulants in hot water, and remove him to bed.

"In all cases of apparent drowning, continue your efforts for at least two hours, or until the responsibility is shifted upon a physician.

SUFFOCATION FROM GAS.

"Usually caused by ordinary illuminating gas, but sometimes by the vapor produced by burning charcoal in a closed room. In these cases the patient is suffering not only from want of oxygen, but from poisoning of the blood, produced by absorption of gas. The heat of the body is not lost to the same extent as in drowning.

"*Treatment.*—Give fresh air. Open all doors, and raise or break windows from the outside, if possible. If not, open the door, cover your mouth and nose with a towel wet in water, or water and vinegar. Rush to the nearest window, break a pane, thrust your head out, and take fresh breath. Repeat at the other windows. As soon as possible remove the patient to fresh air.

"1. If the patient is breathing, slap the

chest with a cold wet towel, or pour hot and cold water alternately on the bare chest. Let him inhale the fumes of ammonia, or burn feathers under the nose.

"2. If the patient is not breathing, perform artificial respiration.

"Wrap a hot plate in a towel and lay over heart. As soon as the patient can swallow, give stimulants in hot water.

POISONING.

"A poison is any substance which, if taken internally in sufficient amount, will cause death. As a matter of practical importance, poisons are divided into two classes, irritants and narcotics.

"Irritant poisons are substances which will corrode and burn the skin or flesh with which they come in contact; for example, strong acids and alkalies. In other words, they destroy, to a greater or less depth, all the tissues of the body which are touched by them. The effects of an irritant poison are evident immediately after it is taken. The symptoms consist of a burning pain in the mouth, throat, stomach, and abdomen, followed by nausea and vomiting. Faintness and shock are also present in varying degrees.

"On the other hand, in narcotic poisoning, the symptoms come on more slowly. Take an overdose of laudanum, for example. It is a preparation of opium. After taking it, a period of fifteen or twenty minutes will elapse before any effect is perceived. The person then begins to be drowsy. The drowsiness gradually increases, until it results in a profound sleep or stupor, from which the patient can be aroused with difficulty, if at all. This shows the difference in the two kinds of poisoning.

"With irritants the effects—pain, vomiting, and shock—appear immediately.

"With narcotics the effects—usually drowsiness and stupor, no pain—are comparatively slow in making their appearance.

"There are some substances which have both irritant and narcotic properties, in different proportions. In poisoning from such substances, the symptoms are of a mixed character.

TREATMENT OF POISONING.

"1. If you know the poison and also its antidote, give the antidote at once. An antidote is a substance which will either combine with the poison to form a harmless compound, or something which will have a directly opposite effect upon the body, thus counteracting the influence of the poison. After administering the antidote, the case falls under the following rules:

" 2. If the poison is known and its antidote has been given; or

" If the antidote is not at hand, and procuring it would cause delay; or

" If the poison is unknown;

" Cause vomiting as quickly as possible, so as to remove the poison from the stomach. The means by which this may be accomplished are as follows: Stir in a tumbler of water a tablespoonful of mustard or salt, and make the patient swallow the whole. It will usually be quickly rejected, bringing the contents of the stomach with it. Two or three teaspoonfuls of the syrup of ipecac will have a similar effect. If none of these are at hand, compel the patient to drink lukewarm, or even cold, water until vomiting occurs. If the case is one of attempted suicide, it may be necessary to open the mouth by force, and keep it open by inserting between the teeth a cork, or the handle of a table-knife. Then thrust the finger down the throat, and hold it there until the patient vomits.

"After vomiting has been caused, you should give to aid it, and also to protect and soothe the walls of the stomach, one or more of the following substances: milk, uncooked white of egg stirred up in water, flour and water mixed, gruel, boiled starch, or oil. The last should not be given in phosphorus poisoning.

SPECIAL POISONS AND THEIR ANTIDOTES.

"This list includes only the more common poisons.

"ACIDS.—Nitric, muriatic or hydrochloric, sulphuric, and oxalic, excluding carbolic acid.

"*Antidotes.*—Baking soda, a teaspoonful in a cup of water. Lime water, as much as the patient can swallow. A teaspoonful of magnesia, whiting, chalk, tooth-powder, or lime scraped from a plastered or whitewashed wall, stirred into a cup of water. A tablespoonful of strong soapsuds.

"ALKALIES.—Lye, soft soap, various washing fluids and powders, strong ammonia, or hartshorn.

"*Antidotes.*—A tablespoonful of vinegar in a cup of water. The juice of two lemons, with an equal quantity of water. The juice of two oranges may be given, if the others are not at hand. Acids and alkalies combine to form harmless salts, or, in other words, they neutralize each other. Oils—olive or salad, linseed or castor—form harmless soaps.

"ARSENIC.—Some rat and fly poisons.

"*Antidote.*—A preparation of iron freshly made. Send to nearest druggist for 'antidote to arsenic.'

"CARBOLIC ACID.—This is not a true acid.

"*Antidote.*—There is no chemical antidote. Give oil freely, olive or salad, linseed or castor.

"IODINE.—The most common preparation is the tincture, or 'iodine paint.'

"*Antidote.*—Boiled starch. Laundry or corn starch, arrow-root, boiled or baked potatoes.

"LEAD.—Sugar of lead in some lotions and hair dyes. Paint containing white lead.

"*Antidote.*--Epsom salts, a tablespoonful in tumbler of water.

"MERCURY.—The most common poisonous preparation is 'corrosive sublimate,' used to kill insects, and as a disinfectant.

"*Antidote.*—Uncooked white of egg forms a comparatively harmless chemical compound.

"OPIUM. — Common preparations: morphine, laudanum, paregoric, many cough medicines, and soothing syrups.

"*Antidotes.*—Opium poisoning is so common that it is more fully noticed here. There is no chemical antidote for opium; but strong coffee, pain, and motion counteract its effects. The patient may breathe very slowly; the pupils, or round dark centres, of the eyes will be very small—the so-called 'pin-hole pupil.'

"Give with the emetic, or as soon after as possible, large quantities of strong black coffee. Keep the patient awake by forced walking. Whip the back and legs with a light cane, or a slipper, or strong twig, so as to produce a smarting pain. Dash cold water on face and chest at intervals. Finally, if the breathing becomes very slow, only five or six times per minute, perform artificial respiration.

"PHOSPHORUS.—Some rat pastes which have a strong odor. Matches.

"*Antidote.*—Common turpentine, which has been exposed to the air for some time, mixed with magnesia. Send to druggist. Do not give oil, as it favors the action of this poison.

"SILVER.—Nitrate of silver, sometimes called lunar caustic. Frequently used in solution as a local application.

"*Antidote.*—Common salt. A teaspoonful in a cup of water.

POISONED WOUNDS.

"The term refers to the bites of rabid or venomous animals. Included under this head are the wounds inflicted by the bite of a snake, or a mad dog or cat. Stings of insects are small poisoned wounds.

"*Treatment.*—This must vary in severity and extent, as follows:

"*a.* If the bite is judged to be only slightly poisonous, or, if doubtful,

"(1) Provided the wound is on a limb (finger, toe, arm, leg), tie immediately a string, cord, or handkerchief twisted into a cord, tightly around the limb, just above the wound. This will prevent the entrance of the poison into the circulation, as it cannot pass above the ligature.

"(2) Draw the poison from the wound by means of suction with the mouth. Even the venom of snakes is harmless when taken in the mouth, unless there is a scratch or wound of the lips or mouth.

"(3) Bathe the part freely in warm water, or, better still, an antiseptic solution, preferably carbolic acid.

"*b*. If the bite is known positively to be dangerous or fatal, use the ligature and suction as before. In addition,

"(1) Make a cross-cut through the centre of the bite, with a pen-knife. This will encourage bleeding, which tends to wash the poison away. It also exposes the wound more thoroughly for the next step in treatment, which is

"(2) Cauterization. This measure is, of course, painful, and apparently brutal. It should be remembered, however, that the bite is almost invariably fatal and a human life is at stake. You have a choice of means. The best is the use of pure nitric acid. Dip the end of a match or splinter of wood into the acid, and thrust it repeatedly into the depth of the wound, so as to bring the acid in contact with every part of its surface. Pure carbolic acid may be used in the same way. If these are not at hand, a knitting-needle, piece of wire, or knife-blade may be heated, and the wound thoroughly seared.

"(3) Give stimulants—brandy, whiskey, or wine—in large doses; not enough, however, to produce intoxication. Aromatic spirits of ammonia, a teaspoonful in a wineglass of water, may be given every fifteen minutes.

"If bitten by a dog, do not allow the animal to be killed. By waiting it will be ascertained if the dog is really mad, and many days of anxiety and worry will be spared.

"For the stings of insects, bind on a compress wetted with carbolic solution, or, better, household ammonia."

1. Prof. Laborde of the Medical School in Paris has recently promulgated a new theory of resuscitation in cases of asphyxia, by pulling out the tongue of the patient, grasping it firmly, and stretching it at regular intervals, say every ten seconds, and then relaxing it without letting it go. Now and then the process should be stopped in order to ascertain whether breathing has begun again. In a great number of cases, after a few of these stretchings of the tongue a spasmodic inspiration is said to take place. If a second one seems inclined to follow, or does occur, the aim should be to have a succeeding pull coincide with the next inspiration, and so on until respiration seems to be able to go on of its own accord. It is claimed for this method that it is easy and simple, and may be applied by any one; and that it is even more effective than the usual method of artificial respiration. It is advocated in cases of asphyxia from drowning or any other cause, and of electric shock.

2. Cider vinegar is an antidote for carbolic acid.

3. Since Dr. Butler's book was written, a wonderful antidote for opium poisoning has been discovered—permanganate of potash. It is claimed to have saved many cases apparently hopeless, and seems to work like magic when injected hypodermically. The enema of black coffee is also more efficacious than when it is given the patient to swallow, as the poison which has gone into the system is more quickly reached in this way.

4. Authorities differ on the value of cauterization. This should generally be left to the physician. There may be cases where it is undesirable. The main thing, of course, is to get as much of the poison out as possible.

CHAPTER XXXI

HOME NURSING

> "Nor love nor honor, wealth nor power,
> Can give the heart a cheerful hour
> When health is lost. Be timely wise;
> With health all taste of pleasure flies."

THE home nursing field is quite as broad as that of emergencies; not that we can dispense with the services of the professional nurse—she has come to stay—and the amateur makes no encroachment whatever upon her valued services. Home nursing involves an entirely different phase of sick-room care. It is for incipient ills, emergency nursing, whether of accident, contagion, or the culmination of chronic disease, and for convalescence, which in many instances is a more dangerous period than the acute stage of illness, inasmuch as doctor and skilled attendant usually dismiss themselves, and home folks assume the *rôle* of nurse. The patient is then exposed to dangers of over-indulgence in diet, and too much sociability. Besides, she naturally spares the nurse-amateur all possible outlay of energy, thereby often denying herself attention she really needs, and would demand from a paid attendant. On the other hand, the nurse-amateur often dissipates her strength in care of the sick one, considering it a virtue that she "neither eats nor sleeps;" and the probable result is that both she and the invalid sooner or later need to resort to the sanitarium, that blessed haven of repose for our women who practice every feature of economy except economy of health.

Education in home nursing should include, among other features, a knowledge of human nature, and how to manage emotional natures, so that mental strength may be imparted by every influence. Too many patients are made worse by the emotional attitude of sympathetic friends, who imagine that such influence is helpful. The best of all sympathy is that expressed in strong deeds, with emotion suppressed. There should be no faces present in the sick-room that do not lend cheer and courage. The kind services of neighbors are much better declined than accepted; and even the one that knows "she can cheer the convalescent" would better withhold her ministrations until a sufficiently long period of repose and isolation places the patient in so resistive a condition that fatigue is no longer a continual menace. The human animal, like the dumb brute, needs absolute rest when under the ban of physical pain and its weakening results, and the mind should not be excited by much conversation. The instances are rare when an invalid really thrives on diversion. She is apt to think she does, and to accept all that is suggested to her. She is temporarily exhilarated by it, but reaction of some description is sure to follow. Let the habitual sick-room visitor have this continually in her mind.

Here I can only give suggestions concerning sick-room influences, and in so doing I shall doubtless antagonize many who are serene in the belief that the customs of their ancestors in sick-room care were correct; while, if we will but reflect that a knowledge of the body in their day was chiefly vague conjecture, and that their theories were not scientifically grounded, we will be glad to select such of them only as we find are in accord with nature's plans. The points I shall seek to cover are ably supported by our best specialists.

The sick-room should be bright, cheerful,

airy, dry, far removed from unpleasant odors, sharp or sudden and startling sounds, and other known unfavorable influences. The ground floor is undesirable for obvious reasons. If possible, there should be opposite windows in the room, but care must be taken to keep one or the other shaded, to prevent the nerve-wearying influence of "cross lights." The head of the bed should be toward the strongest light, if possible, although some of our nerve specialists, on account of the polarity of the earth, place it toward the north first, south second, east third, but never toward the west.

Admit as much sunshine as possible; provide screens to prevent inconvenience to the patient's eyes. Sunshine and air are nature's restoratives.

Ventilation should be carefully planned. A current of air is necessary, but avoid a draught on the patient, especially in cases of pneumonia. It may be best in such cases to ventilate through an adjoining room, covering the head of the patient for a few moments, at intervals of an hour, and fanning with the door, to change the air. An open fireplace is of great importance in ventilation, and a fire burning within it helps to draw the current up the chimney. Even a burning candle may serve this purpose, and in summer is preferable to the heavier fire. A window open at top and bottom helps to make a current, and there are many ingenious ways of improvising shields to prevent a draught from blowing directly on the patient. One of the best is to have an open window covered entirely with canvas or canton flannel. The air passes through the material, but without draught. Chill is more generally caused by draughts than by too cool a room, if it is cooled evenly. Chill may contract the pores and check perspiration. It may cause congestion, or it may cool the surface of the body so much as to demand more heat to be generated than the vital functions can supply. A high temperature is bad. Sixty degrees is about right for the sick-room.

A single bed is better than a wider one in case much care is needed, as the nurse can handle her patient more easily. A wide bed is the best when the patient needs frequent change of position. Two sets of bed clothing are necessary, that one may be aired, while the other is in use. Wool blankets are preferable to down or cotton covers. Down is too heating. Cotton absorbs and retains impurities, while wool allows them to pass through its texture. The skin can breathe better through wool than through any other material. Pillows of varied sizes should be provided; soft hair is recommended as better than feathers, as it is cleaner and less heating. Easy springs and a hair mattress are necessities.

The room furnishings should be simple and restful. Always avoid perplexing patterns in wall paper for sleeping-rooms; for such, substitute plain designs and soft tints. Place a table near the bed, but allow no accumulation of bottles thereon. Have poultice apparatus and other paraphernalia within easy reach, but always out of the patient's sight.

Conversation should be cheerful, but neither hilarious nor incessant. Avoid whispering or mysterious actions. Talk your secrets beyond the patient's ear or ken. Only pleasant, even tones should be heard in the sick-room.

Creaking hinges may be cured by an application of soap or oil. Creaky shoes are an intolerable abomination. A stealthy tread is hardly less distracting. So, let the step be firm—it gives evidence of courage—but the foot-gear soundless.

The carpet-sweeper and dust-cloth (slightly moistened) are the only implements of the kind suitable for the sick-room. Fires should be made with as little noise as possible; fuel can be placed in paper bags and laid on, thereby preventing the usual sharp sounds attendant upon replenishing fires.

Prepare foods in small quantities, without consulting the patient, and give only those of a hygienic nature. Miss Nightingale says, "To watch for the opinions that the patient's stomach gives, rather than to read analyses of foods, is the business of all those who have to settle what the patient is to eat—perhaps the most important thing to be provided for him, after the air he is to breathe." Remove the tray as soon as the meal is finished. Encourage, but do not force, the patient's appetite.

I will give here a valuable contribution to this chapter, from the pen of Mrs. Sarah Tyson Rorer of the Philadelphia Cooking School. I feel it is a boon to the home nurse to be provided with a recipe for making a nutritious beef tea, which is entirely different from the worthless stuff too often imposed upon the sick and feeble in the name of sustenance, but in which nearly all the nourishing properties have been destroyed by cooking at too high a temperature, until there is barely an ounce of nourishment left in a gallon of the liquid.

Mrs. Rorer's directions are as follows:

"Chop one pound of beef freed from all visible fat. Pour over it one pint of cold water, and stir thoroughly until reduced to a pulp. Cover the bowl, and stand in the refrigerator for two hours. Then put over the fire in a porcelain or agate saucepan, and stir carefully until it reaches one hundred and fifty degrees Fahrenheit. Remove instantly and strain. Beat the white of an egg; mix carefully with the beef tea. Put over the fire again, and watch every instant. As soon as it clears and separates, strain again through cheese-cloth. Add salt, and it is ready to serve. It may be re-heated as required, but the utmost care must be taken that it does not heat to the point where bubbles form, as that will harden and separate the albumen which it is the object of this method to preserve. By following faithfully these directions, a perfectly clear, reddish-brown liquid will be obtained, which is very palatable, and contains ten per cent. more nutriment than that made by the old-fashioned method."

Drinking hot water between meals (see chapter on Digestion), and accompanying it, in some cases, by stomach rotation, is of much benefit to the digestive organs. If these organs were kept in healthy condition, there would probably be no malaria. Disease germs develop only in unhealthful soil.

In times of contagion the physician examines the tongues of all the members of the family, to determine the condition of the system and consequent liability to the disease.

Disinfectants should always be at hand, whether the illness is or is not contagious. Use them freely. Carbolic acid is one of the best.

Detail in cleanliness is necessary in sick-room feeding—cleanliness in appointments appertaining to foods, and also to the person. Wash the patient's face, hands, and teeth before the meal; and never consider a person too ill to notice detail. The cases are rare when a patient had best be aroused from sleep for food.

The directions mentioned in the chapter on Massage are invaluable in home nursing. Especial care should be given to posture, particularly in the case of children, during convalescence. Children should be kept on their backs, on a firm bed, and frequent massage should be given them. A sitting posture should be approached gradually, using firm support (a bed-rest, folding-table, or inverted chair) for the back, in place of the usual pillows, which allow the crescent shape of the spine, so disastrous to good health and posture in later years.

Many cases of deformity and of weak internal organs are the result of poor posture during convalescence. We cannot be too cautious about this. More massage and less encouragement to sit up will tend to restore our convalescents to complete health—not semi-invalidism, as is so often the result of less careful nursing. It is not the severity of the illness nor of the surgical operation that fills our homes with invalids—our physicians are now skilled to cope with nearly every form of disease—but it is the lack of rational convalescent nursing, of applied hygienic influences in detail, of self-knowledge and self-economy during the days of recuperation; the lack, we may say, of thorough physical education. Let us endeavor to make home nursing and emergency work important features of education for women and girls in every walk of life.

ENEMATA.

The enema is often of great value in home life, even though actual sickness is not present, and the use of it should therefore be studied theoretically, and the abuse of it avoided. Serious disasters to health have in many instances followed its indiscriminate use. Discreetly administered it is often of value in relieving chronic constipation, and also as a bath in case of diarrhœa or catarrh of the bowels. It should never be considered a remedy, but merely a means of relief, a safe scavenger, for giving nature opportunity of reasserting herself.

I will give general directions in this chapter, and these must be adapted intelligently to individual conditions. The physician should first decide if the enema is advisable, and its frequency. He should also give the diagnosis, so that the patient may decide the posture, massage, etc., that should accompany it.

In case of catarrh of the bowels, dryness or inactivity of colon or rectum, or especial need of cleanliness of alimentary canal as an essential in resisting contagion, the following is a valuable formula:

Prepare a two-quart fountain syringe with hot water not much above the temperature of the body; one hundred and five degrees Fahrenheit is a good average, and one hundred and ten degrees Fahrenheit should never be exceeded, except in special cases recommended by a physician. Add an ounce of glycerine to a quart of water. The same quantity of borax is sometimes preferred in place of this, but the glycerine both softens the water and increases intestinal peristalsis, and is less drying to the lining of the intestine than the borax is. Soap should be used only on approval of the physician. Its use is not always prudent, on account of its tendency to cause subsequent dryness of the tissues. Assume hook-lying or knee-chest posture, and allow two to four ounces to enter the rectum. This is merely to moisten the fæcal matter and cleanse that section of the canal. Retain it but a few moments, and then eject it. The colon bath follows this. Assume hook-lying position, and, during the passage of the water into the colon, stroke around the abdomen, from the left groin up to the short ribs, across to the right side and down the right side. This is opposite in direction to one described for constipation (see chapter on Massage). It is for the purpose of conveying the water into the colon. The quantity to be used (from a pint to two quarts) must be decided by the individual. When discomfort is occasioned, it is usually best to conclude the treatment. Continue the stroking for a few minutes after stopping the enema, and before expelling it. It is unwise to retain it longer than to make the cleansing process complete. While expelling it, stroke as for constipation, to help empty the colon. The stroking during the enema will allay the pain usually experienced, but it may be also necessary to occasionally check the too rapid flow of water by closing the fountain valve for a few moments, continuing light stroking.

At best, the enema is contrary to the laws of nature, as nature demands activity toward, instead of from, the rectum; hence the stroking is necessary to aid the work. The laws of gravitation require that we assume a recumbent or knee-chest posture. It should never be taken from sitting or standing posture.

Some physicians recommend the patient to lie on the right side for the colon bath, as gravitation then aids the passage of the water; but the massage I have recommended is preferred by many, as it stimulates the activity of the colon, and also works the water into the sections of it, making the cleansing process the more complete. There are specific cases when lying on the left side is necessary, in order to localize the treatment in the sigmoid flexure; except in such cases the posture is unwise, for gravitation cannot well aid the water in reaching the entire colon.

The "liver bath" is of much benefit to malarial patients, and to those of torpid liver; it also cleanses the small intestine. It should never be given until the colon has been cleansed by the bath above described, as it is unwise to allow the colon contents to be carried back into the small intestine. Lie on the right side for this treatment, as from this position gravitation will take the water around the colon. During the enema, stroke up the right side of the abdomen. The movement tends to open the ileocæcal valve, the one that closes the passage between the small intestine and the colon and prevents the passage of fæcal matter backward into the small intestine. The stroke is not necessarily heavy, but it aids the passage of the water into the intestine. The quantity of water should be decided by the discomfort produced. A pint for some would be sufficient, while others can take two quarts. Rotate the small intestine (see chapter on Massage) after the treatment is completed. The liver bath stimulates the portal circulation, and is usually followed by bile discharges.

In case of prolapsus of the rectum or of the pelvic organs, the knee-chest position is the better for the enema.

Immediately after breakfast is a good time for this treatment, as such duties are in keeping with nature's plan. Rest should follow. Bed-time with some may be a preferable hour.

Olive oil and water may be a necessity; the oil furnishes nourishment, is healing, and softens the fæcal matter without irritating the tissues. It is generally preferred for children in convulsions.

The invalid is frequently artificially nourished by the enema. Beef tea or any predigested food recommended by the family physician should be used for this.

I repeat again, these directions are general, not specific, and the physician should be consulted before adapting them for use.

CHAPTER XXXII

CONCLUSION

"Oh, excellent! I love long life better than figs."
—SHAKSPEARE.

IN concluding this volume I desire to answer a frequently asked question: "Is absolute health possible?" Barring accident and contagion, we may safely say yes, providing the laws of nature are followed to the letter. Even unfavorable heredity can be overcome by this obedience, and longevity induced, often excelling that of the individual of more favorable heredity, who is liable to fall into the error of believing himself possessed of inexhaustible powers, and is therefore indifferent to hygienic rules, in which case ill health is the inevitable result.

We seldom find a person truly observant of health principles until the need of such observance is thrust upon him. The treasury of health is apt to be depleted by encroachments, and then he turns and asks: "What shall I do to be saved?" Fortunate, indeed, is the mortal that, when this stage is reached, hears not the malediction: "Too late; ye cannot enter now."

Even were we, who have learned the value of the human machine, to attain to the best development of its resources, health would still be degraded by the many who would continue to disobey nature's laws, and consequently would bring disease and suffering into our midst. It is, therefore, the solemn duty of every one of us to encourage the masses to study these laws, and to enforce them in our homes and in public. Set a good example, not only for the public good, but for the safety of ourselves and of our families.

We do not need to visit the sanitariums and insane asylums to ascertain the extent of invalidism in our country; look into any and every home. It is there that it is most apparent, and there the remedy should be applied. At home we have conveniences for following all the laws of health outlined in this work, and we can devote ourselves to them with far less expenditure of time and money, and to much better advantage, than by going elsewhere for the purpose. Many persons cannot go to sanitariums, rest cures, or to places for a summer's outing, but all can practice the laws of health at home. This need not be looked upon as a bore, but as necessary education or discipline to prepare one's self for living.

The lessons here outlined are not to be practiced for the purpose of attaining facility in the execution of the movements themselves. They are but the means to the end, which is muscular control, gracefulness, good carriage, harmony of strength, organic health and consequent longevity and usefulness of career.

The thought should not be laid aside when the practice period is completed. It should attend all the details of every-day life; *i. e.*, in stooping, bend from the hips instead of curving the spine; the knees-bend movement may also be employed to lessen the distance. In sitting, observe good leverage always from the lower spine, no matter how unnatural it may at first seem. From such posture no downward pressure of the viscera is occasioned, such as accompanies the careless posture to which reference is made in the chapter on the Spine.

In walking, observe good poise and even carriage, and avoid the careless posture and gait so often habitual with hurried or preoccupied Americans. It is never too late to correct bad habits, but it is much easier to begin right, and then we will not have them to correct. Good posture should always be practiced, and should be as much second nature as the ability to stand or to walk at all.

Sleep eight hours or more, and always in rooms that are continually ventilated. Conditions and environment determine this.

Clothing worn during the day should be aired at night, and *vice versa*. Beds and bed clothing should be aired, and sleeping-rooms should always be well ventilated. Nothing refreshes one more than fresh air, whether at night or by day, and too much attention cannot be given to this. Be a "crank" on the fresh air and exercise question.

Cleanliness should be made a habit; and where our occupations compel us to handle unclean substances, it should be second nature with us to remove the uncleanliness as soon as opportunity presents itself. The morning bath should be a habit from childhood on.

Habits are our characteristics, and can be controlled by the will, if taken in season and the remedies properly applied. If this is not done they merge into mental diseases. Nail-biting, for instance, has been proved by science to be a disease; and an examination of the brains of those addicted to this bad habit has shown abnormalities in the brain cells.

Were the diseases known as "nagging," and the "blues," checked in their incipiency, we would have fewer victims of delusions and of melancholia, fewer monomaniacs, and less insanity. What blissful home atmosphere, were all nagging eliminated!

Avoid disputes, as well as nagging. Giving way to one's temper makes sad havoc with nerve strength.

Indiscriminate kissing is a habit indicative of insincerity.

To see one's mental and moral, as well as one's physical errors, is of great value in self-preservation. This is made easy by reflectively viewing the faults of others, and aiming to avoid them in ourselves. It is extremely ludicrous to hear a woman who is given to exaggerations, talking of other women evading the truth.

Brinton says: "A sincere lover of truth is never wholly in the wrong, chiefly because he never claims to be wholly in the right."

He also says: "People talk willingly about

their physical ailments, but unwillingly about their moral defects; though the former cannot be mended by discussing them, and the latter might be."

Never hunt for offences; never look for trouble. Many anticipated troubles never come at all, and nearly all troubles can be adjusted when they do come.

Cultivate reposeful habits, but shrink from laziness. Success attends deliberation.

Cultivate cheerfulness, and find the best of everything, but not the worst. Almost every walk in life has a bright side, or at least bright points. Find these, and do not lament because you fancy your lot is not as good as another's. He may have a skeleton in his closet of which you little dream. Things are not always what they seem.

Never give advice unasked. It worries you to have it scoffed at. Study a person's likes, and cater to them as far as you consistently can. Do not discuss subjects that you know will be unpleasant to others, but drop such at once, if started.

Always show deference to a guest. If the guest is not courteous in reply, be chary about inviting him next time.

Religion and politics are always dangerous subjects for argument, and gossip is extremely bad form.

Study the Sermon on the Mount. Its teachings conduce to health and long life. By attention to these things, you will attain health, the Mecca of our pilgrimage, and will be a useful citizen, bringing joy and peace and aid to all about you. Age will have no terrors, and at the end you will enter peacefully on the long journey, satisfied that you have made the best use of the powers with which nature has endowed you.

> "Nor love thy life, nor hate; but whilst thou liv'st
> Live well; how long, how short, permit to Heaven."
>
> —Milton.

www.ingramcontent.com/pod-product-compliance
Lightning Source LLC
Chambersburg PA
CBHW032306280326
41932CB00009B/720

* 9 7 8 3 3 3 7 7 2 4 0 6 1 *